MAN v FAT
THE WEIGHT
LOSS MANUAL

D1354474

ABOUT THE AUTHOR

Andrew Shanahan is an award-winning journalist and entrepreneur who runs the world's best free weight-loss magazine for men: **www.manvfat.com**.

From his work writing about food for the *Guardian* and being named one of the country's best young restaurant critics by the *Independent on Sunday*, weight has always been an issue. His recent experience of losing a lot of weight left him stunned about how little help is directed at men who are dieting. Consequently, he launched his new project - **www.manvfat.com** - to help normal blokes who simply want to win their own battle with fat. Launched after a successful crowdfunding campaign which drew support from Jamie Oliver amongst others, MAN v FAT seeks to inspire, motivate and educate men.

MAN v FAT
THE WEIGHT LOSS MANUAL

START SHEDDING POUNDS NOW →

ANDREW SHANAHAN

Dedicated to God.
And to Emma, who is still waiting for her pink toilet.

Heartfelt thank-you to: Harry Shanahan,
Frank Shanahan, Craig Morris, Emma Jones, Mark Milward, Adele
Hartshorn, Vicky Howarth, Mark McGill, Sarah Herbert, Helen O'Connor,
Clare Sheard, Chris Sheard, Yolander Yeo, Clare Hulton, The Amazing
Losers and the future Amazing Losers on the MAN v FAT site,
Muna Reyal and the Headline team.

Copyright © 2015 Andrew Shanahan
The right of Andrew Shanahan to be identified as the author of
the work has been asserted by him in accordance with the
Copyright, Designs and Patents Act 1988.

First published in full colour in 2015 by Headline Publishing Group

First published in black and white in 2021 by Headline Home
An imprint of Headline Publishing Group

1

Cataloguing in Publication Data is available from the British Library

ISBN 978 1 4722 9002 1
eISBN 978 1 4722 2529 0

Designer: Yolander Yeo
Editor: Simon Davis

Printed and bound in Great Britain by Clays Ltd, Elcograf S.p.A.

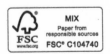

Headline's policy is to use papers that are natural, renewable and recyclable products and made from wood grown in well-managed forests and other controlled sources. The logging and manufacturing processes are expected to conform to the environmental regulations of the country of origin.

HEADLINE PUBLISHING GROUP
An Hachette UK Company
Carmelite House
50 Victoria Embankment
London EC4Y 0DZ

www.headline.co.uk
www.hachette.co.uk

CONTENTS

THIS WAS SUPPOSED TO BE A PINK TOILET...

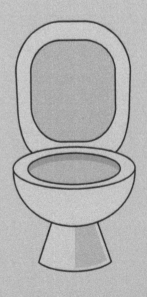

FOREWORD

Back in January of 2014 me and my wife Emma had saved up some money because she had her heart set on a toilet. She's fairly easy to please like that. Frankly, she deserved it. She's the only woman in a house full of men and, without going into too much detail, most of the time even I don't want to share a toilet with us. So she had it all planned, a little extension at the back of the house, a pink toilet, that expensive plush loo roll and absolutely no men allowed. Then MAN v FAT ruined everything.

In June of 2011 I was getting out of bed and I took a 'guttie' – a selfie of my naked gut. At that time I weighed the better part of 231lb (104.8kg). My Body Mass Index (BMI) was 34, I was obese. I had developed a heart rhythm problem due to my weight and I was stressed in my work. I could blame my career writing about food and reviewing restaurants for the likes of the *Good Food Guide*, the *Guardian*, *Time Out* and *Metro*, but the honest truth is I would have figured out a way to get fat regardless of what my job was. I ate crap, drank lager to de-stress and got marginally less exercise than a high-security prisoner in solitary confinement.

The result was the sort of gut that spilled out over my belt, a belly-button you could pothole in and man-boobs that would have driven a 12-year-old girl wild with jealousy. Initially I took the guttie to send to a mate to make him laugh (that's normal, isn't it?) but there was something about the image that made me stop in my tracks. The thing was that as I looked at it I just didn't see me. I saw someone fat and old and miserable. Where was the man who had things he wanted to do? Where was the dad who wanted to run around with his children? Where was the husband who wanted to be attractive to his wife, or at the very least not to nauseate her. Where was I? That guttie provided the shock I needed. I knew I was going to change. I put aside my pride and started to look for help on losing weight.

What I was about to find out was a shock. You see, as a man, the dieting industry had turned its back on me. Despite being desperate for information and support, it turned out that dieting was strictly for women only! How do I know? I know because I read the diet magazines that showed me bikinis that would flatter my figure on the beach this season. I went and sat as the only bloke in the weight-loss groups and listened for an hour about how my period would cause bloating. There was just something about the Diet Coke Man adverts that suggested perhaps I wasn't the target audience. I lost interest.

It dawned on me that the reason I was struggling is because men don't diet, they 'get ripped'. They follow the editorial insanity of men's magazines' promises to give them a six-pack in six weeks. Never mind that at over 30% body fat the only way I could have got a six-pack in six weeks was with surgical intervention, secret NASA technologies and the intercession of a bona-fide miracle. The *Men's Health* world taught me about magical supplements and expensive specialist equipment that looked like it belonged in a Guantanamo interrogation suite but promised me pecs that could dance their way onto a Broadway show if I just kept to the 30-day programme. I lost interest.

The irrelevance of what they were offering left me searching for other answers. I found none. I began to wonder how many other men out there were being led down the same dead end that I was and finding that their hopes to simply shift a bit of weight were being met with the indifference of the diet industry, or the absurdity of the fitness industry. Where was the advice for men who simply didn't want a beer belly any more? I felt that someone had to do something about it – after all, I was just one of 20.4 million men in the UK who were overweight and obese. Around the world there were over 500 million men. Who was helping them?

By making some very simple changes to what and how I ate and getting active (see page 218 for exactly how I got healthier), over the next couple of years I dropped the weight, to the point where today I'm 167lb (75.7kg). I've lost over 60lb (27kg) and I'm back in 32" trousers, which I haven't worn since I was 14. I'm fitter than I've ever been and I'm still eating delicious, healthy food and still enjoying beer, wine, pizza and ice-cream in a 'diet' that I've come to genuinely enjoy. I've started doing triathlons and yoga. My heart rhythm is under control and I'm far less stressed.

When we started making plans to renovate the house I wasn't working. I'd sold my previous business the year before and vowed that I wouldn't do anything until I felt that I had an idea that I absolutely had to work on. Em kept talking about the pink toilet, but my mind kept coming back to all of those blokes who needed help

'Men don't diet, they "get ripped". They follow the editorial insanity of men's magazines' promises to give them a six-pack in six weeks. Never mind that at over 30% body fat the only way I could have got a six-pack in six weeks was with surgical intervention, secret NASA technologies and the intercession of a bona-fide miracle.'

with their weight. One evening, I sat Em down, fed her Guinness and explained that I thought we should put the pink toilet on hold and use the money to launch a magazine for men who wanted to lose weight. I said I thought we should give it away for free and try and make an impact on the lives of the millions of men who currently had no information or support. To her credit she didn't hit me straight away. We agreed to think, talk and pray about it. In the coming days I noticed she'd stopped pinning things to her 'Dream Toilet' board on Pinterest and we both got a really strong sense that MAN v FAT was the right thing to do.

We launched a crowdfunding campaign which hit 102% of its target and drew support from Jamie Oliver and got organisations like the British Dietetic Association, the National Obesity Forum and the Food and Drink Federation supporting it. You may have noticed that sometimes you have to push really hard to get any forward momentum on a project at all – with MAN v FAT we tapped it and the whole thing just kept rolling, crushing everything in its path. Soon we had one thousand, two thousand, six thousand subscribers – the numbers kept growing. The website got tens of thousands of users in the first month alone. We launched the magazine on 5 May 2014 and this book was conceived and agreed by the end of the same month. MAN v FAT is now helping to support and champion thousands of men who want to lose weight. If you're looking for a fresh start, for some guidance, or just for someone to cheer you on in your battle against fat then you've found it.

And it all came from a pink toilet.

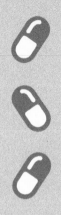

*This book is not
a magic pill.
The act of buying
this book will not
make you lose weight.
But if you follow
the advice you
will lose weight.*

WHAT IS MAN v FAT?

Let's be very clear about what you will get from reading this book:

- Understanding about why you are fat and what to do about it
- Insight into how other men have lost weight using different methods
- Inspiration and motivation
- Help choosing what diet to do, including how to create your own
- Good habits that will significantly improve any weight-loss plan
- Exercise plans that you can start regardless of your size or fitness
- A structure that will help your weight loss succeed regardless of what diet you do
- Tools that will improve and support your weight-loss efforts

One of the biggest issues that men face when it comes to weight loss is that they often diet on their own. Going it alone leads to a lack of structure and support which often results in men creating massively unsustainable programmes. If you've ever written a plan building yourself up to 1,000 sit-ups in a month, or faded after two days on your Only Lettuce Plan then you'll know what I mean. Men often don't feel that they can get advice on a diet, so they cobble together their own plans from bits of advice their mate once read in a magazine. The result is that they have an incomplete system to follow, no structure to make sure it succeeds and their motivation disappears.

If you don't know it, the process of losing weight can take years to get right and all the while you're struggling with it, you're guaranteed to fail at any diet you try. So what is the process? Quite simply it's the three steps that this book takes you through:

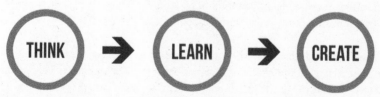

Step One: Understand why you got fat   **Step Two: Learn how to lose weight**   **Step Three: Create a winning structure**

This book will help you master this process. The knowledge that you gain from reading it will ensure that you are equipped with the know-how to control your weight for good.

Let's be very clear about what this book is not:

- **This book is NOT a diet plan.** It will not tell you what foods and drinks to consume to create weight loss. But it will help you choose a diet plan to follow.
- **This book is NOT a magic pill.** The act of buying this book will not make you lose weight. But if you follow the advice it contains you will lose weight.
- **This book is NOT an exhaustive encyclopaedia of weight loss.** The aim is to address the main questions that men have about weight loss.

This book is written by a journalist who has had first-hand experience of weight problems. My skill is a lack of embarrassment at asking smart people stupid questions and presenting the information to you.

I promise that you will not have to purchase any special MAN v FAT equipment, there are no sachets of secret MAN v FAT powders, nor will you be obliged to attend an expensive but secretive retreat once a year – the knowledge of weight loss will be yours to use and freely share forever more.

It should also be noted that this book works from the premise that the reader is coming to this subject fresh. It might well cover some topics in a very basic fashion, or skirt over some of the more in-depth nutritional science. Frankly, I'd rather some readers felt that they were being spoon-fed than leave others wondering which fork they're supposed to be using. Weight loss can be as simple or as complicated as you want to make it. You can understand just the basics and still lose weight perfectly successfully. Alternatively, if you want to read this book and then go on to study fast-twitch muscle fibres and glucose response, knock yourself out!

The other thing that this book will not do is take sides in the senseless and boring diet wars. Research has found that the difference between diets is minimal. People who stick to a diet lose roughly the same amount. The key issue though is that it needs to be a diet that you can stick to – it has to fit with your lifestyle and preferences. Why promote a more expensive high-protein diet if you're on a restricted budget? What good is a juice fast to someone who can't stand smoothies? There are a million different paths that will lead to a fitter and healthier you – this book will show you where they are and help you to choose which one is right for you to follow.

HOW TO READ THIS BOOK

The MAN v FAT book is based on your choices. At every step in the book, you will be making choices and taking actions based on your situation and preferences. That does mean that you have to do some work. Throughout this book are tips, actions and tools for you to use. You will find that a workbook or notepad will come in useful while you are reading the book as there are many times when you can take something away from the book and apply it to your life.

Throughout the book you will see Amazing Losers – normal men who have lost weight using a variety of different methods. All of these men are members of the **www.manvfat.com** site, so if you want to talk to them in more depth about their weight-loss journey, then simply register on the site for free. Search for their name at **www.manvfat.com/members** and you'll be able to connect directly with them.

The book will describe a range of different concepts and use a number of technical terms. Simple explanations of these terms are to be found in the glossary at the end of the book.

Many of the book's resources and tools will require you to access the MAN v FAT website (**www.manvfat.com**), though we've tried to keep the references and web URLs as simple as possible. Alongside the book is the MAN v FAT magazine which you can get on your computer, smartphone, tablet, Kindle or laptop. There's also a forum which provides you access to all the tools and support you could need. This means that with the book, the magazine and the website you already have an ongoing support network for your weight loss.

The one thing that I can't provide is a desire to change your life and to be healthier. I can help improve your motivation, but I cannot (and should not) tell you to lose weight. If you are happy with your weight, and your body and fitness levels do not stop you from doing what you want, then this book is not for you. If, however, you want to beat fat, to live longer and to extract more joy from your one and only life, then read on.

Let's get started.

LES STRATFORD

Age: 45 **Job:** Restaurant manager **Height:** 6'2" (193cm)
Heaviest weight: 511lb (231.8kg) **Lowest weight:** 190lb (86.2kg)

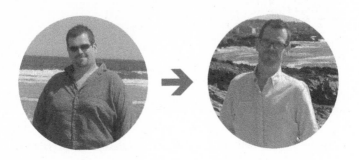

At my heaviest weight I got laid off from a job. About a week later I found I suddenly couldn't breathe, hardly at all. Crazily, I didn't go to the hospital – I went to a birthday party! A couple of days later this was still going on and my roommate said, I think you should go to the hospital. At the hospital they found six huge blood clots in my lungs and later that night I flatlined. I stopped breathing and when I woke up doctors and nurses were standing over me asking questions.

I had to choose between a risky surgery or a medical coma – I took the surgery. They had to strap up the fat from my stomach and pump chemicals into my lungs to bust the clots and after about half an hour of this I could breathe again. Lying on that operating table I was epically obese. I had a 64" waist and I was tearing through 5XL shirts. I was mammoth. I stared at the bright light above the operating table and said, 'OK, seriously dude, if I make it through this I am going to get fit in my forties, because what the hell have I done?'

I was always obese as a child – I thought I was big boned and I just accepted that. Back in the early 90s I dieted and got down to about 250lb (113kg) but then I had a bad accident at work. At that same time a relationship I was in ended and those two things just got me. I spiralled after that. I pretty much spent the next 17 years not caring, right up until I flatlined. It was suicide by food. Occasionally, there would be something in my head saying, 'What the freak are you doing?' Part of you would be trying to wake up and change, but the other part of you is like: whatever.

When I first got home from the hospital I decided to get active by walking more, but after the surgery they weren't sure if there was lung or heart damage. So until I had a follow-up appointment I was a real wuss! I'd walk three-quarters of a mile away from home and come back. I also started monitoring what I was eating. I wasn't counting calories per se but I was starting to push sweets away.

When I started walking I was a snail! My knees hurt and I had an ankle I'd sprained a couple of years ago that would lock. In some ways I felt lost, yet I was incredibly focused, so I was no longer sitting down and playing a video game when I came home, I was researching what I should be eating. I do all my own cooking now and I always keep a food diary. I look at some of the things that I used to eat and shudder. My 'diet' was mostly reducing carbs and avoiding sweet foods. From there it was all just good improvements to my diet, better snacks and hydrating properly.

I still love walking but now I do an insane amount. My shortest route is 4.3 miles, but on a day off it's anywhere between nine to 11 miles, I can do 4.3 miles in 58 minutes. Now my legs don't get fatigued at all. Once I got under 300lb (136kg) I joined a gym because I wanted to try and get a little bit of strength and muscle and burn more calories and now I go three times a week.

It took a long time but I lost the weight and my health is back to normal. The biggest difference for me now is that my whole mental picture is incredibly optimistic. When I was at my heaviest I'd just play *World of Warcraft* but now I wonder if I can get my 4.3 miles done! If you want to lose weight you should know that it's absolutely possible. Believe in yourself and love yourself, because I clearly did not. Know that you never stop learning or progressing, and enjoy the fact that the journey never ends, although it nearly did for me!
www.manvfat.com/members/les-stratford

KIERAN ALGER

Age: 36 **Job:** Journalist **Height:** 5'11" (180.3cm)
Heaviest weight: 184lb (83.5kg) **Lowest weight:** 164lb (74.4kg)

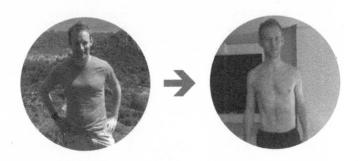

My weight loss was goal-orientated which made it a lot simpler. I had run the
London Marathon before, but I really wanted to run it in under three hours and
I decided I was going to do anything I had to in order to achieve that. I'd always
been a footballer until my early 30s but then I got into running in a big way.
I carried a bit of weight around my stomach, but generally I thought I was pretty
healthy: I loved fruit, I didn't eat any junk food or fried foods. Like a lot of
runners I ate a lot of pasta and bread for the carbs. My treats were beer and very
milky lattes with two sugars. I was running a huge amount but I never really
seemed to lose any weight, I had a body fat of 15% but the fabled six-pack was
nowhere to be seen.

All of that changed when I had a meeting with Giuseppe Minetti from PaleoGym.
co.uk, who was one of the trainers for an event I was doing. He put me through
some resting metabolic rate and fitness tests. I honestly thought he'd say I was the
perfect example of an amateur athlete! What he actually said was that I had the
metabolism of a 50-year-old obese man and that if I stopped running I'd balloon
up within a month! He said that if I wanted to hit my target of a sub-three hour
marathon then I'd have to change the way I ate to a paleo-inspired plan. The rules
were simple: no sugar, no gluten, nothing from grains, no legumes, no dairy.

I switched almost overnight to a diet of lean protein, leafy greens and vegetables, limited fruit and about an 80% reduction in my alcohol consumption.

I don't think he thought I'd follow the rules as strictly as he'd suggested but I was brutal. I wouldn't use an OXO cube because it had gluten in! Porridge and blueberries were out for breakfast and instead I ate spinach, poached eggs and salmon or ham. Lunch was a mixed salad with protein and dinner was vegetables with protein. I worked on the theory that my plate would be 75% vegetables and 25% lean, quality protein. Snacks were mixed raw nuts. It was an expensive diet but very quickly I began to see a difference. Within a fortnight it felt like someone had deflated my stomach and I was already down a notch on my belt. My running improved immensely – I was shocked how much more freely I could move as the weight came off. I felt more energised as well and for the first time I started to approach the weights section of the gym. I'd always been a bit fearful of it before, but now I felt like I had the energy not just to run but to lift as well.

You might not feel like you're carrying a huge amount of extra weight – I didn't – but there are still huge benefits to be gained from addressing what and how you eat. I think from an active point of view the energy that I have from losing the weight and really fuelling my body properly is astounding – it gave me a new lease of life. I felt my body tighten up and grow stronger – it was such a positive thing. The weight loss was in many ways a nice by-product of addressing what I ate. When I was out with friends they'd ask whether I was miserable cutting out all of these things, but I didn't feel like that, ever. If anything I was more engaged with what I was eating. I found new recipes and started to learn how the food I ate not only impacted on my performance as an athlete but also on my performance in life.

The three things that had the biggest impact for me were definitely cutting out sugar, reducing alcohol intake and cutting out gluten. Those things really work. I thought I'd miss dairy the most, but I didn't really miss it at all. You very quickly adapt and you reap the benefits from those changes. When I came to the race I was confident that I'd done everything I could to prepare. I'd trained hard, lost 20lb (9kg), built lean muscle mass and my body fat was down to 8%. I finished the race in 2 hours 57 minutes and 56 seconds. Next year it's the Marathon des Sables!
www.manvfat.com/members/alger-kieran

STEP ONE:
UNDERSTAND
WHY YOU GOT FAT

SKIP THIS STEP IF:

- You know what causes men to get fat
- You know precisely why you gained weight
- You have taken all the necessary steps to ensure you've changed

*'I'm not overweight,
I'm undertall'*

Anon.

SPOILER WARNING:

You are fat because you took in more calories than you needed. In short, you've been eating and drinking too much and you've not been moving enough to offset the incoming calories. That's it. That's why you're fat.

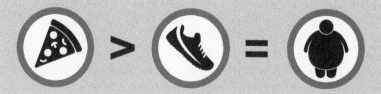

CALORIES IN > CALORIES OUT = FAT

The body is a very effective machine, but it's a real doom-monger. It is always planning for what happens if everything goes wrong; for when the days of feasting and plenty disappear and the famine comes again. Consequently, one of the prime directives the body has is to try and avoid any energy passing out of the system. Instead it takes that excess energy and stores it in handy fat form across certain regions of your body.

We see this across the animal kingdom – a natural programme that allows for rich times and fallow periods. Think of the lions who sometimes get lucky and come across a big elephant carcass they can have an amazing feed on. Delicious. The problem comes when you realise that at other times you can't find an elephant carcass for love nor money. Fortunately, the canny lion's body has stashed some of the energy away in the form of fat. So, for now, the lion doesn't die. Result.

The problem in the human world is that excess calories lie in wait at every turn, but your grumpy body doesn't know that you're unlikely to face much in the way of starvation. Pessimist that it is, it's still storing those extra calories away, saving the energy for a day when the supermarket shelves are bare and you start to get hungry.

The additional problem for modern humans is that we rarely forage and hunt across great expanses of the world to track down our food any more. Instead we drive to the supermarket and push a trolley around, or sit still and do an online shop. Someone else does the hunter-gathering stuff for us, so the extra calories keep coming, you burn off very little and your body keeps stashing the excess energy away. One day you look in the mirror and realise that you jiggle a lot more than you remember.

What's fantastic about this knowledge is that it really doesn't matter who you are, how old you are, how rich you are, or where you are in the world – this fact is true for you too. Take a look at anyone who has their own battle to wage against fat and it will apply to them. To get rid of the fat, you just have to reverse the process. Take in less energy than your body needs and force it to make up the balance with the fat from the bank of energy you keep in your gut.

Frankly, you could stop reading this book now and you would be equipped with the basic knowledge that you need to go away and change your life, win your battle with fat and keep it off forever.

And yet...

And yet, understanding the basic concept of something isn't the same as having a detailed working knowledge of that thing. I can sit in my garden and watch planes flying overhead with a general idea that the miracle of flight is something to do with thrust, wing shape and drag, but put me in the cockpit of a 747 and pretty soon you'll have 500 passengers who are keen to find someone with a bit more understanding of the concept.

So now we understand what's happened to you, let's forget about the WHAT and work out exactly WHY it happened.

'MAN v FAT is not pushing a commercial diet. I want
you to beat fat and then go and live a long and healthy
life in complete control of your weight. To do this
we have to start at the beginning – we need to look
at what your poison is when it comes to incoming energy
and, more importantly, to discover why you are
poisoning yourself.'

Why you are fat is probably a question that you've asked yourself before; if not, ask
it now: why are you fat? What combination of events and circumstances led to your
body being swollen with that weird, yellow gunky stuff we call fat? In many cases
it's not a particularly simple question. For me I was eating and drinking the wrong
foods in the wrong quantities, but I was doing that because I was stressed with a
working situation that meant I was doing stupid hours and then 'rewarding' myself
with crap, instant-energy foods. I added to the problem by sitting motionless all day
in front of a computer and because I was already fat I opted out of any activity that
came my way due to embarrassment and fear. The only thing that allowed me to get
out of that situation – the stress, the food, the lack of activity – was developing an
understanding of what was actually going on.

In every man's battle against fat, understanding what got you into this mess is
essential if you are to get out of it and not simply repeat the same mistake and
put the weight back on again. It's a strange characteristic of the diet industry that
commercial diets spend very little time wondering what caused you to gain weight.
Cynical types might suggest that there's very little value for companies to keep you
at your goal weight forever. It's always better to have repeat customers, isn't it?

MAN v FAT is not pushing a commercial diet. I want you to beat fat and then go and
live a long and healthy life in complete control of your weight. To do this we have
to start at the beginning – we need to look at what your poison is when it comes to
incoming energy and, more importantly, to discover why you are poisoning yourself.

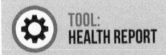

TOOL:
HEALTH REPORT

Go to **www.manvfat.com/healthreport** where you will find an in-depth questionnaire about your health. Here you can answer some questions about you and your habits anonymously and get a detailed analysis of the state of your health. If you've ever had questions about your weight, your fitness and how healthy you are then that is precisely what the Health Report is designed to give you.

The Health Report will give you:

- Your suggested weight targets and BMI (see page 158)
- Your current health
- Your chances of developing various weight-related conditions
- Your basal metabolic rate (see page 74)
- Your activity levels and what you need to improve on
- Your hydration levels
- Your sleep levels
- Your digestive health

The report will also show how you compare to an average person of your age and suggest a number of changes that could result in a healthier lifestyle.

OUR SURVEY SAID...

If you want to know what makes men fat then there is a very useful pool of people to ask: fat men. So that's exactly what we did. We launched the Big Fat Survey – an extensive questionnaire polling the views of thousands of overweight and obese men around the world. This gave us one of the most detailed pictures of men's weight issues ever assembled. One thing we looked at was the reasons why men get fat in the first place. The results were surprising:

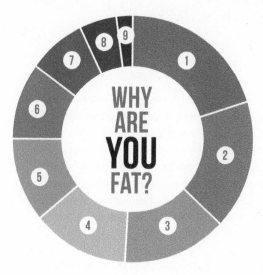

1. **TOO LITTLE ACTIVITY OR EXERCISE**
   20%
2. **MOTIVATION**
   17%
3. **STRESS**
   14%
4. **CAN'T CONTROL APPETITE**
   13%
5. **METABOLISM SLOWING DOWN**
   11%
6. **LACK OF KNOWLEDGE**
   10%
7. **TOO MUCH ALCOHOL**
   8%
8. **LACK OF SUPPORT**
   5%
9. **NO IDEA**
   2%

Over the next section we're going to look at these reasons in more detail and explain what to do if they apply to you. Along with your Health Report (see previous page) this will give you insight into your own situation. It's likely that your own circum will have more than one of these elements at play and, in fact, it may involve all of them.

1 TOO LITTLE ACTIVITY OR EXERCISE
Chosen by 20% of men

IN YOUR WORDS

- "I'm stuck at my desk all day, then sat on a train home, when I get back there's no time left to exercise."
- "I haven't been running for 10 years, not sure I could start now."
- "I've got a bad knee so exercise is out."
- "I'm so tired from work I don't have the energy to exercise."
- "No time, no energy, no chance!"

SUMMARY

Let's look at what constitutes being active. In the UK the guidelines are that you should get 150 minutes of moderate exercise (defined as exercise that noticeably raises the heart rate) every week, in blocks of more than 10 minutes. One way of looking at it is to say that this is five blocks of 30 minutes. In the Health Survey for England only 66% of adults were meeting these levels. This was self-reported, so it's likely that the actual number is much lower – in our survey 52% of men reported getting two hours or less of exercise per week. Certainly from our survey, it was the most commonly cited reason for gaining weight – clearly this is a big issue that needs solving.

From a biological point of view inactivity is bad because you are missing the opportunity to burn up calories, which means you put on weight. A lack of exercise also means that your metabolism slows down and you will find it harder to burn through the calories you consume. On top of that inactivity is a killer – increasing your risk of coronary heart disease, cancer, depression, stress, dementia... there is pretty much no condition that exercise won't help. Of greater relevance to your battle with fat is that with exercise you can burn through the calories you consume.

COUNTING CALORIES

3 pints of Stella
= 745 calories
= running
for an hour
at 5 mph

**1 thin slice of
white bread**
= 50 calories
= 50 press-ups

**Half a bag of
plain crisps**
= 100 calories
= standing at your
desk for an hour

6 oranges
= 300 calories
=60 minutes
of walking
at 3 mph

170g of ham
= 260 calories
= 60 minutes
on the driving
range

300g of chicken
= 651 calories
= 60 minutes
of swimming
front crawl
at a slow pace

All values approximate and based on the energy expenditure of
a typical 205lb (93kg) man.

IS THIS AN ISSUE FOR YOU?

Ask yourself: do you get 150 minutes of moderate exercise per week? If not – why not? What are the reasons you give when it comes to why you avoid exercise? State them here:

I don't get 150 minutes of exercise per week because:

1. _____

_____

2. _____

_____

3. _____

_____

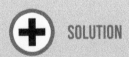 **SOLUTION**

We've covered this in great detail, with solutions on how to get anyone into exercise regardless of your current fitness levels or how much you loathe activity. Turn to page 104 and find out how to work around any excuse you can conjure up.

HOW DO YOU GET ACTIVE WITH AN INJURY OR DISABILITY?

There are a number of medical and physical conditions and disabilities that can impact on your weight. For men some of the most common are hyperthyroidism (an over-active thyroid), Cushing's syndrome (caused by a tumour of the pituitary gland) and perhaps most relevant of all: chronic stress (see page 33). Equally, many men who were active earlier in their lives have injuries – often quite debilitating ones – which make them wary of starting a new fitness routine.

Even if you have a medical condition that doesn't immediately affect your weight gain then it could be that the medication you take for a condition could be making it harder for you to lose weight. Anti-depressants, beta-blockers, heart medications: all of these common medications will have side-effects such as weight gain or a reduced metabolism, meaning that your battle against the fat just got harder but – and this is vital – not impossible.

TIP *If you are disabled, carrying an injury or being set back in your weight loss by a medication, speak to your doctor and get a plan for what to do about it. Do not accept being fobbed off. Find another doctor, a better consultant – keep going! You may have become so accustomed to the fact that you have a bad knee or a messed-up back that you have accepted the idea that there is nothing that can be done about it. Yes, it's harder to lose weight if you are injured, disabled or ill, but it doesn't mean that it's impossible. The simple truth is that if you want to achieve it and you reach out for support then you will find a way – and if you keep looking you will find someone who can support you.*

2 MOTIVATION
Chosen by 17% of men

IN YOUR WORDS

- "I just can't be bothered."
- "When I'm on a diet I get bored and then stray."
- "I don't need to lose a lot of weight, so it's hard to get too worked up."
- "I start loads of diets but they never last longer than two weeks."
- "I find it really hard to stay motivated on a diet."

SUMMARY

17% of our survey respondents said that this was the reason they were fat. The comments given showed that motivation is a diverse issue with many different facets. All of them seemingly come back to 'truths' about dieting:

1) Going on a diet is going to be hard or miserable
2) Diets require massive and sustained willpower

Fortunately, both of these truths refer to short-term or extreme diets. Of course it takes a lot of motivation to only eat lettuce and carrots all day. If you do that then your body will rebel and you will spend your life thinking and dreaming about food – usually extremely calorie-rich foods.

IS THIS AN ISSUE FOR YOU?

Do you find yourself falling off diets after a week or two? Do you know that your weight is higher than it should be but you struggle to get too worried about it? Do you simply think that dieting is not worth the effort and you're actually OK with being fat?

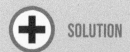

SOLUTION

Forget about BMI and height/weight charts and answer this very simple question – does your current weight and state of fitness allow you to achieve everything you want to do in life, to the best of your ability? If the answer is yes then no wonder you have a motivation issue – you're happy with where you are! Stay as you are and enjoy your life – read more about the Healthy at Every Size movement and stop reading books about weight loss. If the answer is no, then you have all the motivation you need, but you need to learn to lose weight in an enjoyable way (it can happen – see Step Two) and to plan your weight loss properly (see Step Three). You might also benefit from a bit of a motivation supercharge.

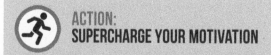

ACTION:
SUPERCHARGE YOUR MOTIVATION

Right now you have a burning desire to lose weight. It might have been a picture, a comment from a colleague or a health scare that set this in motion, but the key is that right now, that feeling is burning hot. As humans we're not designed to keep that level of feeling that high forever. These things slowly cool and eventually we might be able to look at that original motivation and feel relatively calm about it.

We're going to pre-empt this calming of emotion and supercharge your motivation. The best way to do this is to pick three things – three negative and three positive – and list them (see overleaf). The negatives are things that you want to move away from during your weight-loss journey. The positives are things that you want to move closer towards.

→

Examples of negatives

- Doctor warning regarding weight
- Not being able to go on rides at theme park
- Can't walk up stairs without wheezing

Examples of positives

- Able to play with your children in the park
- Looking good in new clothes
- Joining a running club

It doesn't matter what these are – all that matters is that they are relevant to you and that they mean something about what you want to move away from and move towards. The aim is to carry these motivations with you. They should be a daily reminder of where you were and where you are going to be. Be creative and make sure that no matter what you do at least once a day you're going to get a reminder of why this weight loss is important to you.

- Add these onto a small card and keep it in your wallet
- Set a recurring calendar reminder to flash your motivations every morning
- Add these into the tracking book or app you've chosen to use (see page 183)
- Add these onto your gym bag or your workout gear
- Give a copy to the people (see Step Three – page 180) whom you are going to be accountable to
- Find pictures that give you motivation. Again look for images that are both negative – the ones you want to move away from – and positive – the ones you want to move towards.
- Add your pictures as the contact picture for the people who call you most regularly
- Make the pictures your desktop and phone wallpaper
- Get these visual reminders into as many places as you can think of – pin them to a noticeboard, the fridge, the snack cupboard

3 STRESS
Chosen by 14% of men

IN YOUR WORDS
- "I'm stressed looking for work, until I get that sorted I'm stuck."
- "Working long hours and family commitments leaves me with no time."
- "I'm always knackered after work."
- "I want to lose weight but there's too much going on."
- "Stress is the diet killer for me."

SUMMARY

Let's just assume that your job requires that you work long hours and that the amount of pressure you have to shoulder is enough to crush a medium-sized horse. Sound about right? Sadly, you're not alone – 80% of men say that their jobs stress them out. In fact, if you're not stressed you're something of a unique case. But just because workplace stress is endemic it doesn't mean that you should just shrug and get on with carrying your burden.

You should at least understand that long-term exposure to stress does terrible things to your weight and health. When you are under stress your adrenal glands produce more cortisol, the stress hormone. Cortisol is largely responsible for blood pressure regulation and insulin release, and consequently dictates the speed of fat and carbohydrate metabolism. Guess what – all of those factors are related to your weight!

Stress situations also lead to reactions – we try to deal with the stress in our lives by relaxing, which in our culture often means eating, snacking, drugs or alcohol. Guess what – all of those things impact on your weight!

Additionally, more pressure at work often means longer hours, which can impact on your energy levels, sleep patterns and time available to exercise. Guess what – that impacts on your weight too!

IS THIS AN ISSUE FOR YOU?

Some of the classic symptoms of stress are:

- Picking up lots of colds and flus
- Insomnia
- Palpitations and rapid heartbeats
- Headaches
- Upset stomach
- Irritability and anger
- A feeling of losing control or being overwhelmed
- Feeling low self-esteem
- Constant worry
- Low sexual desire or performance

Unfortunately, one of the classic issues with men and stress is that we deny that we are stressed. Whether because we want to protect those around us from feeling that we don't have control of a situation, or simply because we don't want to admit to ourselves that we are under too much pressure.

As a result nothing is done to change the situation causing the stress and it grows from there. If any of this is ringing a bell with you then understand that you are risking your health and jeopardising your weight loss all because of a situation that is absolutely solvable.

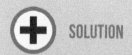 ## SOLUTION

First we have to understand two things.

1. STRESS IS A PART OF LIFE AND NOT ALL STRESS IS BAD

It becomes a problem only when we come under high levels of stress for a prolonged period.

2. WE ALL REACT TO STRESS IN DIFFERENT WAYS

A situation that crushes one man might leave another unfazed. Our reactions to stress also change at different points in our lives. Although you can choose your approach to your stresses you do not get to decide what your body's reaction to it is.

If you are aware that you are under stress that is damaging your health then your first step should be to make an appointment to discuss the situation with your doctor. They will be able to assess your problem and provide a range of solutions. After that, there are three things you can do to take control:

1) Look at improving or removing what is causing the stress in your life.
2) Look at the range of things you can do to help your body cope – these include meditation and breathing (see page 142), getting more quality sleep (see page 134) and improving your nutrition and activity (see Step Two).
3) Recruiting support – whether that's a partner, friend, HR department at work, manager, therapist, local group or online support system.

People under stress often require a lot of convincing that any of these changes will help in THEIR circumstances. Again, this is simply a manifestation of the stress you are under. If you direct your energy at this issue you will discover that you can improve the situation and start to free yourself from the constrictions that chronic stress puts on your life.

SELF-ESTEEM, ANXIETY AND DEPRESSION

There's a slightly misleading view that depression is the common cold of mental health. It's misleading because colds are a communicable disease and they tend to clear up under their own steam (often with the help of steam actually). The same is sadly not true of depression or self-esteem issues.

What is comparable is that both the cold and depression are common. Incredibly common. Over one in four of us will suffer from a mental-health issue over the course of a year. Tragically, suicide is still one of the leading causes of death for men under the age of 35 – we are chronically rubbish at beating this. There's also research to suggest that weight issues and depression are very closely linked. In short, your battle against fat could have a far wider impact on your overall health outlook than you first imagine.

TIP *Talk about it. Either speak to a doctor and get referred or go straight to an accredited counsellor and get help for your problems. Check out www.manvfat.com/resources for online resources to help anxiety, self-esteem and depression. These can be accessed in secret if you don't want to tell anyone. Until you get on top of this then your self-esteem, anxiety or depression will usually find a way of making sure that any positive changes you attempt to bring into your life will be drowned out by a sea of negative thoughts that make progress seem impossible. With help you can absolutely beat this. And once you've learned to beat one foe, the fat won't stand a chance.*

4 CAN'T CONTROL APPETITE
Chosen by 13% of men

IN YOUR WORDS
- "I can never face eating the small portions they want you to eat on a diet."
- "I love food too much to diet."
- "I find I graze all the time, with snacks, finishing the kids' dinner – anything!"
- "I'm always hungry anyway so the idea of dieting is not an option."
- "Snacks are my downfall."

SUMMARY
There's a sexist generalisation that men are either hungry, horny or asleep, and while it's not quite as simple as that, we have to acknowledge that there is some truth in it. In part this is because men DO need to eat more than women – they have taller bodies, a naturally higher muscle mass and therefore they require more energy to sustain them. A very basic generalisation states that an average man will need 2,500 calories per day whereas a woman will need 2,000 (but make sure you take our Health Report to see what your actual daily calorie requirements are).

Over time this extra requirement for energy has come to be seen as a masculine trait. Men who eat more are considered to have a 'manly' appetite. When they're growing up, boys are fed big portions and reassured that they're just healthy, growing boys. In short, we've come to equate mass consumption with manliness. Combine this with the massive availability of food in modern society and the widely held idea that weight loss can only be achieved by an extreme diet that requires deprivation and you begin to see why over-eating is such a big issue for men.

IS THIS AN ISSUE FOR YOU?
Do you find yourself constantly grabbing snacks? Are you often to be found in front of the open fridge wondering what to eat next? Do you hoover up any leftovers on anyone else's plates around the table? Do you constantly think about food?

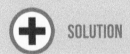 **SOLUTION**

Unlike more involved problems like stress or motivation, solving overeating is largely a question of re-educating your eating habits and getting some understanding of what a 'normal' portion actually is. There are five ways you can solve this and still lose weight:

1. HYDRATE PROPERLY
See page 139. Unless you are getting enough water then your body will keep sending messages to your brain that it needs to consume – often these messages can be interpreted as a need to eat, when really what your dehydrated body is crying out for is liquids!

2. RESEARCH DIETS THAT ALLOW YOU TO EAT UNLIMITED FOODS
Many diets allow you to consume certain foods as much as you like. These are often foods like fruit and vegetables, but other diets allow you to eat as much meat as you like (see Step Two). By choosing one of these and re-educating your snacking habits to avoid calorie-rich foods like sausage rolls, cakes and biscuits you can eat big meals and still lose weight.

3. EAT AT REGULAR INTERVALS
Skipping breakfast is likely to be one of the reasons why you are constantly hungry. Eat three meals a day with two healthy snacks in between and you should find that your hunger is more controllable.

4. EAT SLOWER
It takes approximately 20 minutes for your body to send signals of fullness to your brain. If you are a quick eater or you eat other people's leftovers, then it could be because you are not allowing your body time to send the message that it is full to your brain. Read about mindful eating (page 138) and start to recognise what being full actually feels like.

5. DIFFERENT FOODS HAVE DIFFERENT IMPACTS ON YOUR BLOOD GLUCOSE LEVELS

Foods that are high in protein, high in fat or are slow-release carbohydrates have a higher satiety rating and will leave you feeling full for longer, meaning that your need to snack will diminish. Foods high in simple carbohydrates will not leave you full, meaning your brain will urge you to eat again sooner!

TIP *Different diets define the make-up of an appropriate portion in very different ways. Some argue that you should fill up on fats, vegetables and proteins – others say that's madness and that it's all about eating more veg, lowering fats and boosting carbohydrates. Don't worry – Step Two will cover all of this for you, but it's worth noting that almost everyone thinks that getting more fruit and vegetables is a good idea.*

Currently five portions of fruit and veg a day are recommended, and this would include:

- *Small fresh fruits – two equals a portion*
  (e.g. two kiwis, two satsumas, two plums)
- *Medium-sized fresh fruit – one equals a portion*
  (e.g. one apple, one orange, one banana)
- *Large fresh fruit – half or a large slice*
  (e.g. half a grapefruit, large slice of pineapple)
- *Vegetables – a good rule is four heaped tablespoons equals a portion*
  (e.g. carrots, spinach, broccoli)
- *Salad vegetables – roughly a palm-sized amount equals a portion*
  (e.g. cucumber, tomatoes, celery)

Potatoes don't count. Sorry.

5 METABOLISM SLOWING DOWN
Chosen by 11% of men

IN YOUR WORDS
- "I'm big boned."
- "I eat the same as I did when I was 30 but now I put on weight."
- "My metabolism makes it hard for me to lose weight."
- "Our whole family has a slow metabolism."
- "I seem to gain weight really easily but lose very slowly."

SUMMARY
It's so tempting to blame all of our weight issues on our parents. They were fat, so genetically it's much more likely that we'll be fat. Or to point to a mystical, never-medically-proven 'slow metabolism' for the extra pounds we carry.

To some degree this even has a hint of legitimacy to it. It has been discovered recently that there are genetic markers that make you more liable to be obese but they are only markers, they are not your destiny written in stone. As for your metabolism, you are absolutely right – as you get older your metabolism *does* slow down – but despite what you might have been led to believe, it's not the case that you are destined to get fat at any age.

IS THIS AN ISSUE FOR YOU?
- Do you believe you come from a 'fat family'?
- Were you always overweight when you were growing up?
- Have you told yourself so many times that you are destined to be obese that you now hold that as a firm belief?

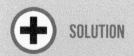 **SOLUTION**

Snap out of it! You are responsible for yourself and your actions – they are what make you fat, not your genes or your metabolism. You are the only person who controls what goes in and out of your mouth (and if you're not then you need to contact the relevant authorities). Genetics and metabolism simply change the terrain of the battleground, not the battle itself. If fat has the upper ground then that means it has a tactical advantage, but it doesn't mean that you surrender. It means you have to understand how to even things up and get on with it.

In the case of your metabolism, it means learning how to optimise it as much as possible. For instance, if you think back to when you were younger and your metabolism was magically faster, you were probably also a lot fitter and carried more muscle. As we age our muscle tone naturally decreases, but it doesn't disappear!

Here are three things you can do to keep your metabolism speedy:

1. KEEP HYDRATED
See page 139

2. EAT REGULARLY AND GET ENOUGH PROTEIN IN YOUR DIET

3. EXERCISE MORE AND BUILD LEAN MUSCLE

6 LACK OF KNOWLEDGE
Chosen by 10% of men

IN YOUR WORDS

- "I never know what diet to do."
- "I don't know how to cook."
- "I don't know any good recipes so I eat the same thing and get bored."
- "I change diets all the time and never find one that suits me."
- "I don't know how to lose weight."

SUMMARY

This is a tough one to admit to ourselves especially, as men, we're sworn to uphold the sacred oath that we shall never admit when we don't know something. Stopping and asking for directions is for women – we'll plod manfully on and figure it out eventually – sound familiar? In many ways it's no surprise that men lack knowledge when it comes to cooking – after all, it's never really something that's taught to us. Even if you love cooking, men often drop home economics as a subject as soon as possible to avoid being the only guy in the class. So we're left to figure it all out as best as possible.

Consequently, a lot of us are left not knowing whether coconut oil or olive oil is more calorific, how we can make vegetables taste delicious and why protein makes for a brilliant snack. This problem often comes into force when men are living on their own and are suddenly responsible for their own cooking, potentially after having a partner or mother to cook for them. Suddenly, they are forced to rely on cheap take-away foods, ready-meals and plentiful snacks to get them through the day – all of which only ends in Fat winning the battle against Man.

The other side of this issue is when you don't know what diet or healthy eating plan to follow. None of the information about diets is ever really focused on men, so we're left to decide for ourselves. We also don't get a good supply of quality information about what constitutes healthy eating – again, we're left to figure it out for ourselves, which inevitably results in men falling through the cracks.

IS THIS AN ISSUE FOR YOU?

- Do you find yourself changing diets?
- Can you make a number of healthy and delicious foods?
- Do you have a good idea of what a healthy diet looks like?

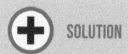 SOLUTION

Of all the issues that cause men problems with their weight, this is the one with the simplest solution... learn!

Give yourself a head start by browsing the recipes at the end of this book, which equip you with enough knowledge to put together a day's worth of healthy meals that can fit into a range of different diets. You can achieve any of these recipes regardless of whether you know one end of a mixing bowl from the other.

If you want more, get on the web – **www.manvfat.com** is a good place to start. If you're still stuck then you could also consider some of the healthy food-delivery companies that bring all of the ingredients you'll need for a week's worth of meals to your door – they'll even cook healthy meals, all you have to do is reheat. And if you want more information about what diet to go for then Step Two will take you through it from beginning to end.

7 TOO MUCH ALCOHOL
Chosen by 8% of men

IN YOUR WORDS

- "I enjoy a drink at the weekend too much to diet."
- "I don't want to give up beer!"
- "There are no good low-calorie drinks for men."
- "Booze kills diets for me."
- "It's not the alcohol, it's eating crap when I'm drunk and hungover!"

SUMMARY

Understanding why you're fat requires honesty. Booze, along with stress (which often goes hand-in-hand with alcohol), is one of the main causes of fat in men, though few of us will admit to it being a problem. Alcohol – and alcoholism – has such a stigma attached to it that we're desperate to avoid anything that makes us think we are in any way abnormal in our drinking. Often we benchmark those around us and say, 'At least it's not like I'm in the pub every night like X'. Or we look back and say, 'But I'm drinking less than I used to do when I was 20.' Sadly, this is a flawed perspective. As a society – especially in the Western world – our alcohol consumption is outrageously high, which is one reason why alcohol-related illnesses like cancer and dementia are so prevalent. We've been swigging with abandon from the boozy teat for too long.

There's a tendency among blokes to look at the Government-recommended drinking levels and guffaw at how eye-wateringly far we over-shoot them, often in one sitting. We shouldn't. We should accept and understand that drinking four units – just over a pint of strong lager or two small glasses of wine – really is the maximum for a day and anything in excess of that constitutes binge drinking. Scary, isn't it? Take a look at the full guidelines:

- Drink no more than 21 units of alcohol per week.
- No more than four units in any one day.
- Have at least two alcohol-free days per week.

A good way to work out the units in alcohol is to look at the strength of what you're drinking. If a lager is 5% then that means it will have 5 units of alcohol per litre of that drink. If you're drinking a 500ml can then that means you're consuming 2.5 units. A shot of a 40% spirit – 40 units per 1 litre bottle – means 1 unit per 25ml shot.

Of course your weight isn't the only thing that alcohol will affect – your liver, heart, kidneys, bowels, fertility and mental health are at real risk of damage when you drink too much. And yet we keep necking it, looking around us and quietly thinking, 'It's not like we'll all die of booze, is it?'

IS THIS A PROBLEM FOR YOU?

Take a look at the healthy drinking guidelines opposite, then ask yourself, do you break them on a regular basis? If so, then alcohol could well be an issue in both your future health and your current weight situation.

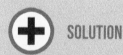

From a weight-loss point of view you need to understand that alcohol is a poison and when you take it in your body prioritises processing and eliminating it, in preference to working its way through the fat cells you'd rather it was annihilating. In short, not only does it top you up with calories, it temporarily stops you from burning through them too. Setting aside the health implications of binge drinking, there are three approaches commonly used by men to solve the age-old dilemma of 'How do I lose weight and still drink?'

1. GO COLD TURKEY

If you're feeling particularly strong-willed or you're not someone who likes to drink then one option is to go cold turkey and cut out alcohol altogether.

Don't fancy that? How about...

2. DRINK AS PART OF YOUR CHEAT MEALS

If you don't care about the consequences of binge drinking and just want a couple of good sessions of boozing per week then you might prefer a diet that has a cheat day or a number of cheat meals built in. See Step Two and pick one of those diets.

And if that's not an option, how about...

3. REGULATE YOUR DRINKING

Most diets allow for moderate consumption of alcohol. As an example, a calorie-controlled diet could incorporate daily drinking but still allow for weight loss.

DRUGS AND WEIGHT LOSS

Although we've covered alcohol, many of the same facts apply to illegal drug consumption and weight loss. Namely:

- Your body has to eliminate toxins from drug consumption
- Drugs and snacking go hand-in-hand – one study put the additional daily calorie consumption for people stoned on marijuana at an extra 600 calories
- Drugs often mean a reduced desire to exercise or be active

Although some studies have shown that drug users (including those who smoke marijuana) often have a lower BMI than those who don't, it's evident that using illegal drugs for weight loss has a raft of issues and should be avoided – even so-called slimming drugs like amphetamine or ephedrine.

If you feel that your alcohol or drug consumption are no longer under your control then speak to your doctor. You are one appointment away from being connected to a world of support and assistance.

8 LACK OF SUPPORT
Chosen by 5% of men

IN YOUR WORDS
- "My girlfriend does most of the cooking and she doesn't want to diet."
- "I don't help myself."
- "I'm my own worst enemy when it comes to diets."
- "We go out a lot with mates and it's very difficult to say you're not drinking."
- "It's hard to stick to a diet when your Mrs is eating a Chinese in the same room!"

SUMMARY
The Big Fat Survey showed that the majority of men felt they got all the support and encouragement they needed (see page 177). But that still leaves a significant proportion of men who feel that there are some serious diet saboteurs around. As much as we might not like to think of our partners as wanting anything but the best for us, we can all be motivated by some rather nasty emotions when it comes to weight. Jealousy and resentment can mean that you don't get the support you need when it comes to losing weight. 'Feeders' – people who get enjoyment from fattening up other people – do exist! If those around you are often saying that they prefer you with some meat on your bones, or insisting that you eat thirds and fourths of their Sunday dinner, then it could be time to start looking at how those relationships impact on your weight.

Are you the fat one in your friendship group or family? Has it always been that way? Do you get referred to as Big Lad? Chunky? Tiny? It could well be that, because your role in your group has always been defined in part by your size, your friends won't necessarily support your decision to lose weight. Largely, this will be motivated by their own fear – if you're not going to be the 'fat one' in the group, then will it suddenly become them? It's far easier to keep you fat than it is to think about shifting a few pounds themselves. Finally, the most common person cited in our survey as giving a lack of support was the person themselves – whether this was as a result of failing to keep to diets, acts of self-sabotage or simply through being annoyed when they made a mistake on their weight-loss journey.

IS THIS A PROBLEM FOR YOU?
Do people support you? Do you find yourself trying to persuade people that what you want to do is a good idea? If you explained your weight-loss plans to people around you, what would their reaction be?

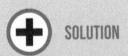 **SOLUTION**

It shouldn't need saying but the people around you should love and support you. This also shouldn't come as a shock to you, but you should also love and support yourself. If you explain what you're trying to achieve and why, then their reponse should be to get on board with your choices. If not, then they might well have weight issues of their own which are interfering with the correct response, which should be a hand-stinging high five and a cry of 'You're going to smash this diet! Let's jog to work together!' To identify where your support and threats come from in your weight loss, turn to Step Three and learn how to build a team of supporters for your diet – including yourself.

'Are you the fat one in your friendship group or family? Has it always been that way? Do you get referred to as Big Lad? Chunky? Tiny? It could well be that, because your role in your group has always been defined in part by your size, your friends won't necessarily support your decision to lose weight.'

EMOTIONAL EATING AND FOOD ADDICTIONS

'Mens Sana In Corpore Sano' – or a healthy mind in a healthy body – is surely one of the ultimate ambitions for any human being... and yet the two so rarely go hand-in-hand. If something is out of order with your mind then your body often suffers, and when things are wrong with our physical health they often impact on our mental well-being. Take comfort from this: beating fat will do a huge amount to restore any self-esteem that has ebbed away. Not only that, but addressing any issues you have with food will also help you to identify and start to solve other underlying problems that exist.

EMOTIONAL EATING AND DRINKING

If you're a fully fledged bloke then the idea that you're reaching for the Doritos because you're sad should be enough to make you laugh yourself daft. It's an absurd concept, isn't it? But at one time or another all of us fall into the trap of thinking that a beer or a chocolate bar will make us feel better. Emotional eating is defined as any time you consume not because you're hungry or thirsty but to deal with another feeling. Sadness, fatigue, boredom, grief, happiness, anxiety, anguish, frustration... To a certain extent it doesn't matter what emotion it is, it's more about the fact that, rather than accepting that emotion and trying to understand where it comes from and how you can deal with it, you eat or drink instead.

Ever found yourself stood in front of the fridge just picking at things because you can't think what else to do? That's emotional eating. Ever been really annoyed with someone and suddenly found that you've whittled your way through an entire pack of biscuits? Emotional eating. It's so endemic that we all do it. It's a simple displacement behaviour – rather than confronting the emotion we channel it in another way.

If it's so pervasive, how can we stop emotional eating? Well, we can't. There will always be days when we are tired or bored and we snack on something or grab a drink that isn't entirely healthy. The key is to see this behaviour for what it is. You might not be able to stop it but you can deepen your understanding of why you're doing it and over time find ways to reduce it. Let's say you constantly find yourself wading through tubs of ice-cream because your manager has overlooked you for a promotion – you need to look at why that is happening to you and solve that problem rather than trying to treat the frustration it causes with treats.

Similarly, food addictions are formed when the feel-good emotion released by the brain when we eat something calorific becomes a drive in itself. The cycle of eating and feeling good is compounded by constant reinforcement and eventually addicts are hooked on getting their fix of feeling good. Food addictions are real and can give men a difficult challenge to overcome when it comes to weight loss. If you worry that you may have a food addiction or any other form of eating disorder then the next step is to get help – check out the organisations at **www.manvfat.com/resources** and see how they can help you get free of damaging behaviours.

*Now we know
why you got fat,
let's learn
how to shift it.*

WAIRA MUNGAI

Age: 21 **Job:** Fitness entrepreneur **Height:** 5'9" (175.3cm)
Heaviest weight: 270lb (122.5kg) **Lowest weight:** 185lb (83.9kg)

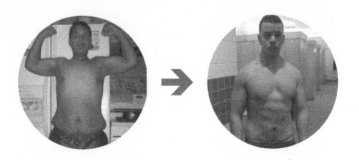

I grew up in a culture where eating was a fun thing, it was what we did when it was a celebration. My family always ate fried foods, heavily processed foods, high-sugar foods and a lot of very big portions. With a father figure in my life I possibly would have been overweight anyway, but because he was gone there was a hole I was trying to fill. I was unhappy from a young age. As I grew up, food numbed those feelings. I tried to get instant gratification with food. At home a typical meal would have been chicken, fried steak, mashed potatoes and gravy, and it would be two big plates. Coming home from school I'd eat half a bag of Doritos. I was drinking a two-litre bottle of pop every day. I was just eating junk all the time.

One morning I was getting a lift to school with my mom and there was snow on the ground. I was getting into the car and I bent over to put my backpack in the car and my jeans just completely ripped. My mom was running late for work so she was shouting at me to get a move on. I had to run inside and in the middle of this snowy, frozen day I had to go to school in the only thing that would fit – a pair of shorts. Walking up to school there was a big glass window and I could see the reflection of my legs in the window. They were just huge and this feeling of sadness and disgust grew around me. That was the moment that I thought, you know what, I don't want to be like this any more. I don't care what it is, I'm going to do something.

Like most bigger guys I had tried all the diets going in the past so I was pretty knowledgeable about how to eat healthily and, importantly, I was finally at an age where I could go to the YMCA and use the gym. So I started going to the Y. That first session I remember I did 25 minutes on the elliptical trainer and that was as much as I could do. I remember leaving the first session and I was dead, I could hardly breathe, my legs were shaking and felt like jelly. But I did it! Then I figured I could do more.

I lost the weight over the summer holidays and back at school people thought I was a new kid. The people who did recognise me went crazy and they would come and talk to me and tell their friends. It was the most uncomfortable feeling I've ever had because as a bigger person I didn't exist – I just wasn't used to being seen. I remember people would look at me and smile and I'd turn around thinking someone was behind me, but it was me they were smiling at. To be completely honest the world is a different place when you're not obese.

If you want to lose weight, first ask yourself why you want to lose weight. If you don't have a strong enough why, you're going to fail when you fall. The difference is, if you have a really strong why you're going to get up again when you fall, and it'll just be a stutter in the journey. You have to be brutally honest with yourself, if it's only about the scales or the way you look then it's going to be tough.

Finally, it's all about submersion. Constantly surround yourself with where you want to go. It needs to become so clear that you can see it in your head. When I was on that elliptical trainer at the beginning I was sweating and panting away, but in my head I had already become the thin and strong person I wanted to be. I had an image of what I looked like taking a girl to the junior prom. And you know what, I made that happen.

www.manvfat.com/members/waira-mungai

CHRIS HORRIDGE

Age: 43 **Job:** Michelin-starred chef and R & D at Ronan Foods Ltd
Height: 5'8" (173cm) **Heaviest weight:** 195lb (88.5kg)
Lowest weight: 154lb (69.9kg)

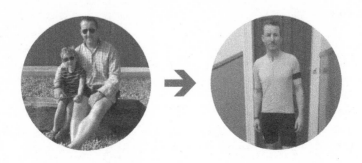

Over my career I've always worked in restaurants and I'd always worked long hours, until I stopped working at my last restaurant. For the first time I actually had night times to myself. I was like, what do you do? What do people do with free time in the evening? So I did what a lot of other guys do, I started drinking heavily! Nothing outrageous, but I'd have a few beers and a few wines in the evening.

One day it suddenly dawned on me that I'd grown out of my 34" jeans and I had bought a pair of 36" jeans and I realised – this is only going in one direction at the moment. At that time I had just gotten into cycling and time-trialling and it's very clear that in that sport it can all be won or lost on a single second. It's about improving absolutely everything, so not just the aerodynamics of the bike and the kit, but also ensuring that the rider is in optimum condition. I wasn't. So I thought I would treat myself as an experiment and see if I could use the science of nutrition to get myself in shape.

I wanted to do this in a very structured, scientific way, so I decided everything would get logged, including what I ate, my training, the sleep I had. I started by working out my metabolic rate and I knew that the difference with me is that I would want to not only lose weight but to be able to train hard while I was doing that. I then created a spreadsheet which very easily allowed me to track precisely what I was taking in and it would calculate what I was getting in terms of protein, carbs, fat and fibre. Everything I ate, I broke down into its constituent parts. So if I had an egg I knew it was about 83 calories and about 7g protein.

Once I'd gone through the ball-ache of creating the spreadsheet it was very easy to add the odd item to it. Then it just churns out at the end of the day what you've eaten and whether you're in a calorie deficit. It also allowed me to make very specific choices about how I got my nutrients. I made sure I was quite high on protein because I wanted to feel full. That worked until the training ramped up and I got to the stage where I did a particular session probably about two to three months in and I ran out of energy in a session – I adjusted my carbs by about 3% and that made the difference. I also wore a Wahoo Heart Rate Monitor during my training so I could track what I was losing.

My weight loss was very solid and predictable and then I got down to 156lb (71kg) and had a bit of weakness. To be quite honest I just thought, 'I've been dieting now for five months, I need a break', but I started eating a bit too much stuff and I put a few pounds on. Then I realised I wanted to get underneath 154lb (70kg). I'm the same weight now as I was when I was 19, only I am actually fitter! What I've noticed is that it's not just my weight, my general health has improved – my skin is good, I feel better, look better, I'm basically bombarding myself with nutrients. People noticed very quickly and mentioned it and I suddenly got smaller trousers. Then the other day I was in the house and Christelle my wife said, 'Bloody hell, you're getting a six-pack!'

If you want to lose weight you need to have a goal. I don't mean weight loss as a goal. It was relatively easy for me because I wanted to be good at a sport so there was another goal – pure weight loss was not necessarily my aim – improving my power-to-weight ratio for cycling was. My goal was to make my cycling better – it made everything so much easier to judge how well I was doing because rather than just the weight coming off I was actually seeing my performance increasing on the bike. Once you see that it makes it so much more satisfying.
www.manvfat.com/members/chrishorridge_

STEP TWO:
LEARN HOW TO LOSE WEIGHT

SKIP THIS STEP IF:

- You understand nutrition
- You know what diet you are intending to do
- You understand how to get back into activity
- You already have a plan about how to get back into the activity of your choice
- You understand all the bad weight-loss habits you should break and all the good weight-loss habits you should make

"What goes up,
must come down."

Sir Isaac Newton

SPOILER WARNING:

You will lose weight by changing the things that you eat and the things that you do. Nutrition and activity – that's it. As with the understanding of why you got fat, this fact is as true for you as it is for the man on the other side of the world, it's true no matter what job you do, how much you earn or how bad you smell.

NUTRITION + ACTIVITY = SUCCESS

Experts like to bicker endlessly about the precise ratio of how important these two factors are but there's some consensus around the ratio of 80% nutrition to 20% activity. I think in the case of men it might be slightly more like 70:30 – because activity and competition for men can be such motivating factors and because our naturally bigger muscle mass means we can shift weight quickly when we factor in exercise – but it's largely irrelevant. The key point is that nutrition – what you choose to eat and drink – is far more important than how much exercise you do.

Why is nutrition more important? It's simple – it's much quicker and easier to consume calories than it is to burn them off. Let's say you hit the gym at lunchtime and beast yourself with an hour-long sprint on the treadmill – depending on your weight you'd be lucky to burn around 900 calories. On the way back from the gym you grab a burger, small fries and medium shake from a well-known burger emporium – total damage 1,300 calories. An hour of sweating, undone by five minutes of eating. It's essential that you understand that any weight-loss programme based only on activity is doomed to failure. You cannot run your way to your ideal weight while eating anything you want. Sorry.

So to lose weight you need to get the **right amounts** of the **right sorts** of foods and fine-tune your body shape by building muscle with activity. That's all it takes. A lot of the confusion about diets comes because what constitutes 'right' for you is a very personal thing. It depends on a number of factors that might be more important to you than the man reading this over your shoulder. Step Two will do the following four things:

- Help you to unravel the confusion about the basics of nutrition
- Help you decide what diet to do
- Guide you in enjoyably improving your activity levels
- Outline good and bad habits that massively impact your weight loss and health

Best of all you get to make your own choices about what is right for you, experiment with that approach and, if you want to, create your very own weight-loss plan.

THE BASICS OF NUTRITION

Let's start with a sad truth: no matter what nutritional approach and activity you choose there will be someone who thinks you're an idiot for doing it that way. They'll pull their faces, exclaim that simply no one is doing low-fat any more and really it's all about ditching sugar and HIT training. By reading this book you can safely ignore these people, who will only be shouting about another trend in a month's time anyway.

Do your own research, learn how to experiment safely with your own metabolism and enjoy the understanding and power that comes with knowing how to get optimum results from your body. You are the one who has the most information about your body and your preferences, which is why you are the one who is going to choose what nutritional approach you take.

TIP *Learn to be as selective with your sources of information on nutrition as you are about the foods and drinks you consume. Even knowing which experts to listen to can take practice; consider the training required to become a...*

Dietician
- *Must be trained to university level or above*
- *Regulated by the Health and Care Professions Council (HCPC)*
- *Term protected by law*
- *Permitted to work in hospitals*

Nutritionist
- *Term not protected by law*
- *Anyone can use the term 'nutritionist' regardless of qualifications*
- *Registered nutritionists must have completed an accredited course*

Diet expert
- *Term not protected by law*
- *No qualifications necessary*
- *No association or organisation*

None of this means that you won't get some rubbish dieticians or a brilliant nutritionist, but it's a point worth noting.

UNDERSTANDING CALORIES

Whether you've been counting calories for years or you are just hearing the word for the first time, it helps to go back to basics. Calories are simply a measurement of the energy that is in any food or drink. They were devised back in the 1800s when Wilbur Atwater burned various foods and measured the energy that was released. One calorie is the amount of energy required to raise 1 gramme of water by 1 degree Celsius (the word calorie is from the French word *Calor*, meaning 'heat'). Atwater's work gave an understanding that some foods contained more energy than others and became a useful tool for understanding weight loss.

To maintain weight, men are advised to consume 2,500 calories per day (women 2,000) and a rough approximation says that 3,500 calories equals one pound of fat. In other words, if you can reduce your calorie intake over a week so that it creates a 3,500 calorie deficit you should lose one pound of fat. However, calories have become increasingly controversial in recent years and it's fair to say that calories alone do not give us a perfect understanding of weight loss. One problem with calories is that it's very hard to accurately measure Calories In against Calories Out (CICO). Nutritional science is difficult because there are so many variables in the human body that it's an imprecise laboratory.

For example, if you burn off 3,500 calories in an epic running session it doesn't automatically mean you will lose a pound of fat – it may be more or less; one of the issues is that you don't just lose fat when you diet, you also lose bone and muscle mass. Add to that the fact that exercise means you will actually gain muscle mass which weighs more than fat and you can see why nutrition isn't a simple science.

Another important consideration when learning about calories is that calories from different sources are not the same, which is often translated into the phrase, 'Not all calories are created equal'. What this means is that depending on the sources of food you eat, there will be different benefits and problems. As we will see, calories that come from protein, for example will result in greater muscle gains.

Calories that are consumed from simple carbohydrates will be converted into energy quicker. Calories from vegetable sources will give you more vitamins and minerals. You may have heard the phrase 'empty calories' before, which refers to calories that are consumed from sources that don't add many benefits to the body. In the ongoing quest for health it's useful to hold on to this concept and make sure that the calories you take in are always doing something beneficial for you.

There's no question that calories give an oversimplified view of energy use within the human body, but they do give us an overall understanding of how fat gain and fat loss occur. It may be that the diet you choose completely ignores calories

'You may have heard the phrase "empty calories" before, which refers to calories that are consumed from sources which don't add many benefits to the body... make sure that the calories you take in are always doing something beneficial for you.'

– that's fine, provided you have an understanding of them. This allows you to experiment with non-calorie approaches but if they don't work for you, you can check your calorie intake and output and get another view on what's going on.

WHY CALORIES COUNT

Jeff decides to follow a raw food diet because it sounds healthy and doesn't require much planning or thinking as his time is short. Every day he eats mounds of healthy foods – cashews, avocados, bananas and pineapples – and washes it all down with whole milk fruit smoothies. After a fortnight he jumps on the scales and is horrified to see that he's gained two pounds. At that point he works out the calories of what he's been eating and compares it to his Total Daily Energy Expenditure (get yours at **www.manvfat.com/healthreport**). He's shocked to find that he's been eating at least 500 calories more than his daily requirement, explaining the weight gain on a healthy diet.

Now that doesn't mean that raw food diets aren't healthy or that calorie counting is always essential, but it does explain why you need calories as an overview. Without an understanding of calories you could find yourself getting frustrated when you follow healthy guidelines and find yourself not just not losing, but actually putting on weight.

WHAT DOES A HEALTHY DIET LOOK LIKE?

If you've done your Health Report you will know how many calories you need to eat to lose weight, so the next step is to decide what to 'spend' those calories on. This is entirely up to you. Let's say that again for dramatic effect: what you eat and drink is your decision. The theory is that as long as you eat and drink within your calorie limits then you will lose weight. One MAN v FAT reader has been tracking his weight loss drinking a bottle of wine every day. He eats very small meals and drinks very large glasses of Malbec. It works for him – even though by his own admission he's hungry most of the time and not particularly happy!

There are three very good reasons why spending your calorie allowance just on lager or McDonald's is a particularly bad idea. That's because the purpose of nutrition is threefold:

TO GIVE YOU HEALTH

The food and drinks that you take in are supposed to create a system of health in your body. Health means that your immune system is strong, you avoid illnesses, and that all of your various biological processes work in the most efficient way possible. Eating for health means that you get a balance of fibre, vitamins and minerals from your food and drink. It means that you hydrate your body well and that nutrients are absorbed into your body with maximum efficiency.

TO GIVE YOU FUEL

Let's never forget that without sufficient food and drink you will die – nutrition isn't optional. However, death isn't the only consequence of poor nutrition – you can also fuel your body so that you never live as fully as you could. If you don't take on sufficient fuel from the right sources of food then you can feel weak, tired and lack drive (of all kinds). Eat too much of the wrong foods and it can lead to weight gain, uncomfortable bloated feelings and lethargy. Fuelling your body in the optimum way means getting sufficient liquids and a balance of foods of different types.

TO GIVE YOU ENJOYMENT

Eating and drinking is one of the great pleasures of being a human. Never lose sight of the vitally important fact that you should enjoy what you consume! If you don't enjoy the diet you choose, you will struggle to stay on it for long. That doesn't mean

'If you don't take on sufficient fuel from the right sources of food then you can feel weak, tired and lack drive (of all kinds). Eat too much of the wrong foods and it can lead to weight gain, uncomfortable bloated feelings and lethargy.'

that the foods we take in can't be both healthy and delicious, but we should accept that some of our calories can go on foods that are from 'bad' sources! As long as those 'bad' sources are in suitable proportion to the 'good' then you will still be able to lose weight.

THE MYSTERY OF THE MACROS

When you look at the majority of modern diets they will often work around promoting a different balance between the three main macronutrient groups (sometimes called just macros) and this is where the war of the diets really begins! The Eatwell Plate promoted by the NHS suggests that you should be eating a low-fat, high-carb diet with some protein and lashings of fruit and veg. However, other diets suggest nearly the exact opposite with high-fat, low-carb diets and more protein. So who is right? This is something you get to decide for yourself – it's possible to lose weight using nearly any method providing the calorie deficit is there so experiment for yourself!

You might think this is a minor issue but the millions of blog posts, tweets and research papers suggest otherwise. The noise around the macro discussion can get very annoying and is sometimes difficult to avoid – the best suggestion is to experiment with the approach you feel best fits your lifestyle and see how it works. With time you will discover a balance that works for you. Just remember that the more extreme a diet encourages you to be is directly related to how hard it will be to follow. I did the Dukan diet (which massively reduces the amounts of carbs you are allowed) and survived for four days before feeling faint whilst simultaneously experiencing explosive diarrhoea. That experiment ended pretty quickly for me, but it might be perfect for you – try it!

NUTRIENTS IN FOOD

The nutrients in food come in three main groups (sometimes called macronutrient groups) and two additional but vital extras:

FATS

Fat is the major form of energy storage in all foods. There are three types of fats: saturated (which mostly come from animal sources), unsaturated (mostly from plant sources) and trans fats (primarily created in laboratories). Foods high in fat include dairy, red meat and oils. The body breaks fat down as a slow fuel source and it is also useful in other body processes. Fat has a high calorie content with 1 gramme of fat containing 9 calories.

CARBOHYDRATES

Carbohydrates are a form of energy for the body. They can either be simple or complex, referring to how quickly the body can break them down and get the energy into the bloodstream. Simple carbohydrates include soft drinks, sugar and white bread. Foods high in complex carbohydrates include brown rice, lentils and wholegrain breads. 1 gramme of carbohydrates contains 4 calories.

PROTEINS

Protein is what your body uses to create new muscle tissue. Foods high in protein include meat, fish, eggs and lentils. Protein also adds bulk to any meal and makes you feel full. 1 gramme of protein contains 4 calories.

VITAMINS AND MINERALS

Responsible for nearly all of the correct functions of the body – from eyesight to energy, skin to bones. They are found in high concentrations in many fruits and vegetables.

FIBRE

AKA roughage – the stuff that your body can't digest. As your body can't process it, it works its way through your system and helps you crap! Found in fruit, vegetables and wholegrain cereals.

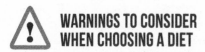

WARNINGS TO CONSIDER WHEN CHOOSING A DIET

SHORT-TERM DIETS ARE NOT AS GOOD AS LONG-TERM HEALTHY CHANGES

There's a good chance that the word diet is one of the most hated in the global vocabulary. Let's be honest, it doesn't get off to a good start when the first three letters spell out 'DIE'. As it happens 'diet' – referring to a short-term radical change to your eating habits – deserves all of the cursing it gets because it is damaging nonsense.

The utter nonsense of short-term diet logic is – 'I'll take a break from my current regime which is causing me to gain weight, switch to an extreme system and endure it for as long as possible.' At that point you generally return to the eating and drinking habits that got you fat in the first place. Guess what happens then? You put the weight back on – and usually some extra, because you're so annoyed that your month of eating rice crackers hasn't worked. People often present that experience by saying that their diet didn't work. Say that enough times and they actually start to believe that they're somehow immune to diets.

Of course quick fixes exist, but you have to accept that if you use them you will be back for another quick fix very soon. The alternative is far more enjoyable – invest time in learning how to change your nutritional and activity habits so that you can live a long, happy life while eating in a way that you enjoy and that promotes health.

BE CAREFUL WITH 'UNLIMITED' FOODS

Some diets have a list of foods that are 'allowed', which are often promoted as unlimited foods. This can be very appealing to followers of a diet because they instantly scan for these foods, stock the fridge with them and eat to their heart's content. The point to remember is that regardless of whether you are filling up on cheese, liver or spinach, if you eat more calories than you need then you will gain weight.

There is a wider point with unlimited foods – men are not cattle. We are not designed to graze continuously. If you consume vast amounts of food throughout the day – regardless of whether it's allowed by your diet or not – then you will start to experience health issues, notably chronic indigestion. You will also find that you are not addressing the deeper problem of emotional eating, when you eat out of boredom, fear or frustration (see page 49).

WHEN A DIET BANS A PARTICULAR FOOD YOU WILL CRAVE IT LIKE NOTHING ELSE

If you've ever been told not to look at something, you'll know that your natural reaction is immediately to stare at it. The same psychological process happens when a diet tells you that you can't eat any given food. You start to crave it out of proportion to how much you actually want it. Be aware that diets that restrict certain foods will mean that you spend quite a lot of your time day-dreaming about eating them. The alternative is to eat everything but with an understanding of the correct portions that those foods should be consumed in.

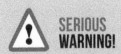

SERIOUS WARNING!

A Very Low Calorie Diet (VLCD) is often described as one containing fewer than 800 calories per day. But if your plan routinely sees you going under 1200 calories then only do so following medical advice. Side effects of VLCDs can be serious – approach your weight loss sensibly.

DIFFERENT DIETS
AND WHAT MEN THINK ABOUT THEM

The Big Fat Survey (see page 25) gave us a clear idea of which diets men are on, and which they are thinking of following. This allowed us not only to build up an idea of which diets are the most popular among men, but also to understand a bit more about the dieting psychology of men.

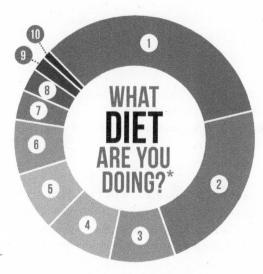

1. **MY OWN RULES**
   34%
2. **CALORIE COUNTING**
   23%
3. **FASTING/5:2**
   9%
4. **LOW-CARB HIGH-FAT**
   9%
5. **PALEO**
   8%
6. **WEIGHT WATCHERS**
   7%
7. **SLIMMING WORLD**
   4%
8. **JUICE DETOX**
   3%
9. **CAMBRIDGE DIET**
   2%
10. **SLOW CARB/4-HOUR BODY**
    1%

Perhaps the most noteworthy consideration is that men feel very isolated from the traditional diets that women pursue – they typically look to follow diets that they can manage themselves. This is probably to be expected after generations of men have been ignored by the diet industry – you can only be bypassed for so long before you decide to work out how to get on with things on your own.

This section should also give you a good idea of some of the different dietary approaches that exist and what your fellow men are doing. Clearly, there is a wider range of diets than the ones described over the following pages so if there is a particular approach that you want to find out about take a look at **www.manvfat. com/diets**. There you will also find the most up-to-date information on these plans as the commercial diets change details frequently.

1 MY OWN RULES
Chosen by 34% of men

IN YOUR WORDS
- "I'm just eating sensibly and trying to exercise more."
- "I hate diets, I'd rather just cut down and try to be healthier."
- "I've got a list of rules that I follow which are common sense but they work."

HOW DO YOU DO IT?
The beauty of following a healthy eating plan that you devise is that you know it fits with your philosophy, because you made it up. It can also be flexible depending on the situation that you are in. It's liberating to know that you are the author of your own nutritional destiny (I should declare my bias here because I followed this approach to lose weight, see page 218).

To follow your own rules, you simply have to create a number of rules designed to create weight loss. The most common comment from men following this plan was that they were 'eating sensibly'. Often the rules included an element of other diets – such as restricting carbohydrates or following a 5:2 plan.

Clearly, one person's definition of sensible will differ from another's, but we can get a sense that it includes some central points:

- Reducing portions and snacks to a sensible level
- Cutting back on 'bad' foods including sweets, biscuits, cakes – this often included reducing bread consumption
- Getting alcohol consumption under control
- Using 'Cheat Meals'
- Eating more 'obviously' healthy foods including fruits and vegetables and reducing processed foods
- Hydrating properly

If you are looking to create your own diet it's important to get a good overall idea of what your body needs in terms of energy and to choose foods that give you a balance of the main food groups (see page 66). Other than that you are free to create the rules yourself and see what effect it has! A general consensus seemed to be that the number of rules should be five or fewer, to avoid getting bored or confused. If you're looking for some ideas for your own rules, read about the other diets and see our list of good and bad weight-loss habits on page 134.

WHAT DO YOU EAT?

Obviously, this depends on your own rules but a typical 'healthy' menu for the day might include: **Breakfast:** Homemade Muesli **Lunch:** Ham and Egg Salad **Dinner:** Thai Green Curry with Chicken. Recipes for these dishes can be found on page 220–2.

WHAT IS BANNED?

Again, what you ban on your diet is largely up to you, although the prime rules concerning forbidden or restricted foods seem to be directed at processed foods, sweets, biscuits, crisps, cakes and alcohol. If you are wondering what to ban or restrict from your 'own rules diet' then these are a good place to start.

IS IT CHEAT FRIENDLY?

Yes. Many men incorporate an element of cheating (see page 136) into their 'own rules diet'.

WHAT MEN SAY
PAUL DOLMAN-DARRALL

I made up four simple rules for myself.

1) Remove bad snacks and drinks from the house. They aren't banned. Just buy one at a time. No multipacks. Consume. Save none for later.

2) 25 minutes exercise, five times a week. No excuses. Always exercise on Monday to kick the week off. I started with fast walking instead of catching the bus!

3) Limit calorie intake two days a week. At its worst this was a light breakfast, lunch and dinner. I aimed for 600 calories but I didn't give up if I went over.

4) Track food intake to improve your choices. I logged my goal with MyFitnessPal and limited my net calories to 10,640 a week (1,520 per day on average). Who knew that just 10g of butter contains almost 70 calories! It meant I saw what was happening with all of my nutritional choices.

I took this approach to minimise the size of the change. I did not want to give anything up. I did not want to suddenly start running marathons. I did not want to change my life but I *did* want to lose weight. Small change, big impact. That was my goal. It has worked so far – 50lb (23kg) lost. It was hard to begin with but creating habits really helps. The other advantage is that it's been very simple to do. It has just involved lots of repetitive, short-term discipline. The only downside is that weight loss is consuming. A lot of my thinking time, concentration, moods and conversations have been dominated by it and it doesn't go well all the time!

www.manvfat.com/members/dolmandarrall

THE MANᵥFAT VIEW

Nowhere is it clearer that men like to take control than in their choices of how they lose weight. Not for them the prescriptive measures of strict diets – they'd rather start with a blank piece of paper and work it out for themselves. This is fantastic and demonstrates a strong resolve. It's also clear to imagine the satisfaction of achieving weight loss following your own system – and it might even be useful for someone else.

The downside is that there is no guarantee that your rules will work. Unless you're creating a calorie deficit then you won't burn fat and this can very quickly become frustrating and lead to your diet being abandoned like the half-built replica of the *Titanic* in the loft. The other downside is that, without a structure in place (other than the one you create), you are far less likely to succeed.

WHERE TO GET STARTED

If you would like to create your own rules diet then this is the perfect book for you. It's full of different tricks and techniques you can add to make up your rules. You could also sound people out about your rules on **www.manvfat.com/talk** and get a second opinion. Another useful starting point (as Paul found) is to closely track your intake and exercise for at least a week so you could see that your system was going to create a calorie deficit. See Step Three to create a winning structure for your rules.

2 CALORIE COUNTING
Chosen by 23% of men

IN YOUR WORDS

- "I'm using MyFitnessPal to track my calories."
- "Simple calorie counting."
- "It's boring, but I'm counting calories."

HOW DO YOU DO IT?

You track what you eat and the total calorie values per day (or per week) so that you eat fewer calories than your body actually needs, forcing it to burn fat. To do this you have to work out how many calories will be too many, too few or just enough for you. Don't use the average recommended intake which would see you getting 2,500 calories per day! A more likely figure will be between 1,400 and 2,000 per day – depending on your current weight, your activity levels and how quickly you're looking to lose weight.

So what is the right amount of calories for you? Fortunately, we have a tool you can use to calculate that – **www.manvfat.com/healthreport**. This will give you a very accurate guide of your BMR and your TDEE:

BMR stands for Basal Metabolic Rate and it's your body's total need for calories in a day. If you just sat on the sofa for an entire day and did nothing but breathe and exist then you would burn your BMR's-worth of calories.

TDEE is the Total Daily Energy Expenditure. Unless you're really lazy then you probably do something other than lie on the sofa all day (get up to go to the toilet hopefully) and the energy that you expend in movement and activity is added on to the BMR to give you your TDEE in the form of calories.

Once you've got your TDEE you simply subtract calories from that total (within safe limits) and you have your very own formula for losing weight. Roughly speaking, 3,500 calories equates to a pound of fat. Therefore if you take 3,500 calories off your total weekly TDEE you should lose a pound. Knock off 7,000 calories and you should lose two. Remove 10,500 calories and you'll drop... you get the point.

WHAT DO YOU EAT?

Anything, as long as you track it. A typical daily menu might include: **Breakfast:** Porridge **Lunch:** Mackerel and Rice **Dinner:** Chilli con Carne. Recipes for these dishes can be found on page 222–4.

WHAT IS BANNED?

Although nothing is actually banned with calorie counting you may find yourself amending your choices to include low-calorie versions of foods – a can of a diet fizzy drink has 0 calories, whereas a can of a normal fizzy drink has 140 calories.

IS IT CHEAT FRIENDLY?

No. All calories have to be accounted for – but that doesn't mean that you can't create a greater deficit during the week with some lighter days and exercise and then use some of the accumulated calories to have a good Friday night out. Provided you create a 3,500 calorie deficit then you should still lose a pound.

WHAT MEN SAY
JOHNNY MORRIS

Losing weight is all about the numbers, isn't it? Well, no. It's about the synergy between all the things you do to burn fat: exercise or the gym, curbing your bad habits and getting enough sleep. You have to get all those under control to really melt the fat away. My take on calorie counting is that it's just another tool, but it's a very good tool. I use calorie counting as a motivator and to keep things in check when my brain tells me, 'Another portion won't do any harm!'

The majority of us have smart phones and to do this right you absolutely have to use an app. In my opinion MyFitnessPal is the best out there purely for its huge database of foods and ability to scan bar codes. I've dropped 60lb (27kg) in five months by counting calories. You do hit a point where you plateau, then things become more complicated as your body adjusts to this new regime so you have to trick it, which is why I think – if you choose to have one – your cheat day is as important as any other day. Pizza is my carb of choice.

The best thing about losing the weight this way is that it hasn't been hard and it's focused me on going to the gym and working harder and harder each time. The worst is the looks I get from my wife as I record everything that goes into my mouth – she thinks I'm obsessed but the trade-off is worth it.

www.manvfat.com/members/johnnytype2

THE MAN ᵥFAT VIEW

One of the real joys of calorie counting is that nothing from avocado to zucchini is off the menu, as long as you keep track of the calories. Provided you aim to eat a balanced intake of all the food groups and don't just spend your calories on chocolate it's a good way of ensuring you get a truly balanced diet. Another bonus is that by tracking the calories you've burned during exercise you can earn extra food and drink which gives you a good incentive to get active. It also doesn't hurt that it's free!

The biggest criticism of calorie counting is that it does require some effort on your part to accurately record your calories. This means faithfully recording the calories from the tomato ketchup to the slice of cake you had at work. Lose track of those calories and mysterious and frustrating weeks of maintaining can begin. Initially, this will also mean that you will have to weigh out foods (at least for a couple of weeks) until you learn to discern 100g of chicken (219 calories) from 250g (548 calories). You also have to have some willpower (or planning acumen) so that when you hit your limit you understand you go bust and stop consuming.

WHERE TO GET STARTED

Get some kitchen scales and choose a system to record your calorie intake as well as a method of working out how many calories are in your foods. Some of the favourite methods of doing this are with apps such as MyFitnessPal or websites like WeightLossResources.

3 FASTING/5:2

Chosen by 9% of men

IN YOUR WORDS

- "I'm trying out fasting."
- "5:2 because it's easy to remember!"

HOW YOU DO IT?

The 5:2 diet is a form of fasting diet, which relies on calorie restriction to create weight loss. Fasting has also been shown to have a number of other benefits including improving digestion and increasing testosterone production – which helps with building lean muscle mass. It's pretty much one of the simplest diets going – on five days out of seven you eat what you want (although dieters are often unclear whether this means you can eat as much as you are physically capable of on these five days – it doesn't) then on two 'fast' days of the week you restrict your intake to 600 calories. By doing this you create a shortfall of around 3,500 calories – meaning you can lose around a pound a week.

WHAT DO YOU EAT?

A typical daily menu for the restricted 'fast' days might include: **Breakfast:** Boiled Eggs and Asparagus **Lunch:** Miso Soup **Dinner:** Cod Fillet and Cauliflower. Recipes for these dishes can be found on page 224–5.

WHAT IS BANNED?

As this is a calorie-controlled diet, nothing is banned, provided you stick to the relative calorie limits on the fasting days.

IS IT CHEAT FRIENDLY?

Yes.

WHAT MEN SAY
ANDREW MALE

I started 5:2 as a New Year's resolution and it's lasted most of the year.
Initially I gained weight because I eat all the time and I *like* to eat all the time.
I can be quite disciplined, though, so I thought that for two days a week out of
seven I should be able to cut down. That's what attracted me to it – it wasn't
something that I had to do every day.

I chose Monday and Thursday for my fasting days because I was at work and
it wasn't a weekend. On the remaining days the theory is you can eat what you
want. Surprisingly, though, you don't gorge yourself. I thought on the Tuesday
and Friday I'd be starving and ready for a massive breakfast, but I didn't feel
hungry at all. One of the advantages of the diet seems to be that it makes you
consider what you're eating at other times.

By fasting I've lost about a stone and a half over the course of the year and I've
lost a lot of weight off my stomach. It's not really been a struggle at all. I've
noticed that my desire to snack has gone almost completely – I still eat big
meals but I don't find myself thinking I need to have a piece of cake with a
cup of coffee or tea.
www.manvfat.com/members/andrewmale

THE MAN▾FAT VIEW

The 5:2 diet has the huge advantage of being simple to understand and often very
effective. It does mean that you will be required to track your calorie intake on the
two days you are fasting and many choose to count on the non-fasting days too.
Clearly, if you massively overeat on the remaining five days then you will not lose
weight, but one of the advantages of having two days of restricted eating is that it
encourages you to understand that often when we eat we do so not because we're
hungry but for any number of emotional eating reasons (see page 49).

Other benefits have also been attributed to fasting, including increased concentration and a sense of calm. That said, a number of people have also complained that the fasting days left them with headaches, irritability and a reduced desire to exercise. Fitting 5:2 around family or socialising is particularly tricky, so choose your fasting days carefully.

WHERE TO GET STARTED
Pick your fast days, find a system of tracking calories and get going!

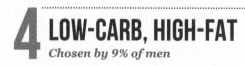

4 LOW-CARB, HIGH-FAT
Chosen by 9% of men

IN YOUR WORDS
- "Atkins appeals because I don't think I'd be hungry on it."
- "Any diet that you can eat massive amounts of cheese has to be good!"

HOW DO YOU DO IT?
The big trend in recent years has been the move towards saturated fat (mainly fats from animal sources) no longer being regarded as the prime suspect responsible for weight gain and instead the blame is falling squarely on the shoulders of carbohydrates, especially refined carbs like sugar. Consequently, many diets have promoted a Low-Carb High-Fat (LCHF) route – among the most well-known is Atkins, while the Dukan diet is similar, though its emphasis is more on the importance of protein.

As you might expect, these diets restrict the consumption of carbohydrates and put more focus on protein and fat as the sources of energy for the body. The aim is to approach a state called ketosis, which is simply the process of your body breaking down fat for energy creation, which in turn produces something called ketones. By eating a low-carbohydrate diet the levels of ketones in the body should be high enough that they are detectable in your urine. Some diets measure this by testing the urine for sufficiently high levels of ketones.

WHAT DO YOU EAT?

Not many carbs! A typical day's menu might include: **Breakfast:** Healthy Fry-up **Lunch:** Greek Salad **Dinner:** Lamb Steak with Yogurt and Harissa. Recipes for these dishes can be found on page 226–7.

WHAT IS BANNED?

Although not strictly banned, carbohydrate consumption is massively decreased. This means that breads, pasta and beer are often the first to go.

IS IT CHEAT FRIENDLY?

Depending on which branch of LCHF you are doing, there are elements that feel like cheating – consumption of high-fat foods is so contrary to the diet advice of the last few decades that eating a steak slathered in brie can make every day feel like a cheat day.

WHAT MEN SAY
SAM FELTHAM

The reason I choose to practise an eat-as-much-as-you-want, low-carb high-fat diet of real foods is because for me it is the most obvious place to start. The randomised controlled trials of the past 15 years show that it is superior to low-fat calorie-restricted diets in helping people lose more weight, become healthier and, most importantly, in keeping more weight off in the long term. What I particularly like about this way of eating is that you do not feel restricted at all. This again has been shown in the randomised control trials in participants' adherence rates and satisfaction scores.

What I don't particularly like about it is how some people make it a licence for literally eating as much as they CAN rather than eating as much as they WANT. Before starting this diet, one should have a full blood profile performed, or at least cholesterol, triglycerides and blood glucose, and then again 30 days later to be sure that it is benefiting your health as well as your waistline.
www.manvfat.com/members/sam-feltham

THE MAN v FAT VIEW

Low-carb high-fat is often popular with men because it's relatively simple – there is no calorie counting or weighing foods out (always a bonus), but you will find yourself tracking carb consumption, which can be a pain. The other huge advantage for carnivorous men is that it practically forces you to eat meat – often for breakfast. This can constitute a big change to the way you normally eat, and although there's no escaping the novelty of burgers (no buns) for breakfast, it often doesn't take long before you start dreaming of Corn Flakes. The meat-heaviness of this diet does also mean that you can struggle if you are a vegetarian – it can also be an expensive way to eat.

It may come as a shock to the system but if you get it right then you can lose weight quite quickly – especially initially. One huge downside is that it can leave you feeling you're missing something – and indeed you are. These sorts of diets are often harder to stick to because there's nothing more guaranteed to start you dreaming about a particular food than the knowledge that it's a forbidden fruit. On which note, it's also worth pointing out that some of the low-carb high-fat approaches also ban fruit.

HOW TO GET STARTED

First of all you need to choose which branch of low-carb high-fat diet you're doing – the main two are Atkins (**www.atkins. com**) and the more protein-led Dukan (**www.dukandiet.co.uk**) – both named after the diets' originators.

5 PALEO
Chosen by 8% of men

IN YOUR WORDS
- "I like paleo because it's simple."
- "Paleo for the meat!"
- "A lot of people at the gym I go to follow a paleo diet and it looks easy enough."

HOW DO YOU DO IT?
The caveman diet is a better explanation of how paleo works (although still a fairly lousy name) because you have to imagine your food being anything that a caveman would have access to – anything you could hunt, fish or gather. This means that you're excluding anything that would be the product of agriculture – for example dairy, grains and legumes (beans and pulses). Paleo also puts an emphasis on the 'paleo lifestyle' which means that it's not just a list of foods and drinks to avoid but a wider creed to fit into your life. A good example of this is that good-quality whole foods are favoured over processed foods – cavemen don't eat ready-meals, remember.

WHAT DO YOU EAT?
The main foods eaten on a paleo diet are meats, salads and fruits (although strictly you should limit high-sugar fruits like bananas, kiwis and mangos.) A typical daily menu might include: **Breakfast:** Eggs and Spinach **Lunch:** Baked Sweet Potato with Bacon and Mushrooms **Dinner:** Roast Chicken with Roast Vegetables. Recipes for these dishes can be found on page 227–8.

WHAT IS BANNED?
Milk, sugar, cheese, breads, pasta, soft drinks, sweets, grains and legumes, fruit juice, peanut butter, all processed foods.

IS IT CHEAT FRIENDLY?

It depends on your take. Paleo fans often rate themselves on just how paleo they are (which can get a bit tiresome), so you might hear people talking about being 80% paleo. The 80:20 approach is quite common – whereby 80% of the time people eat in a paleo fashion, but 20% of the time they stray and indulge in a carnival of bread and ice-cream. As ever, it depends on your own experimenting to see how this affects your weight loss.

WHAT MEN SAY
KEITH NORRIS

My paleo journey began 13 years ago, in early 2001. Frankly, I stumbled upon the health aspects of the diet by accident. Having experience of strength and conditioning training, I knew well the power that carbohydrate manipulation had on body composition in general, and fat levels in particular. But after witnessing first-hand the normalisation of my chronically elevated blood pressure following the elimination of gluten from my diet, I was convinced. A rockin' body composition and superior health? Sign me up!

What's to love about the paleo diet? Well, the most alluring aspect is that it's not a 'diet' so much as an all-encompassing lifestyle. It's not a list of dos-and-don'ts, but a bedrock of scientific principles supporting an over-arching philosophy of superior health and freedom from the 'health-industrial complex'.

In fact, the only thing that I find cumbersome about this lifestyle is explaining the simplicity of the principles/philosophy paradigm to those stuck in the old way of dos-and-don'ts thinking. Paradigm-breaking is hard work!

Is it a simple lifestyle to adhere to? You bet. But simple does not imply easy. At least, not in the beginning. You'll have a lifetime of physical and mental pre-conditioning to overcome, cravings to shake, and habits to break. But after the initial two weeks or so you'll wonder why you hadn't made the change sooner.
www.manvfat.com/members/KeithNorris

THE MAN∨FAT VIEW

Paleo has lots of advantages. It's simple because you're not required to count anything. It also moves your diet towards natural, non-processed foods which have been shown to be better for your health. Depending on your point of view, the fact that it often prioritises meat and fish can be a good thing – although it does mean that it's potentially an expensive diet to follow. Many people find that removing grains from the diet does help with digestive issues – a fact which paleo fans seize on to prove that modern man is not cut out to consume or digest such foods.

As with all restrictive diets that make certain groups of foods forbidden, this can lead to extreme desires to eat those foods (in this case dairy in particular). Perhaps the biggest issue is that as portions are unrestricted it can lead to massive over-eating, especially among men who are perhaps more prone to this than others. This can lead to weight gain – it's perfectly possible to follow a strictly 100% paleo diet and gain weight. If you are eating 3,000 calories per day of meat you will still gain weight, regardless of how cold a shoulder you give cheese.

(→) HOW TO GET STARTED

Get a very clear idea of exactly what foods are allowed and which are banned on the paleo diet. Take a look at **www.manvfat.com/ diets** and you will find a number of resources for getting started with eating a paleo diet.

6 WEIGHT WATCHERS
Chosen by 7% of men

IN YOUR WORDS

- "I like the structure and ease of Weight Watchers."
- "I've lost a lot of weight on Weight Watchers."

- "I do Weight Watchers online."
- "The groups are mostly women but they're welcoming."

HOW DO YOU DO IT?

Weight Watchers is perhaps the world's most famous weight-loss club, spawning the trend for group weigh-ins when it launched in 1963. Everything you put in your gob is given a value (currently called ProPoints) based on its protein, fat, carb and fibre content and you can eat whatever you like as long as you can fit it into your personal points allowance, which decreases as you lose weight. You also get a weekly ProPoints allowance on top of your daily allowance to spend as you like.

Weight Watchers currently offers the Filling and Healthy programme, where you choose freely from a list of unlimited food and use the additional 49 ProPoints spread across the week for everything that's not on the list, which can be handy when you're not in the mood to measure out every single grain of rice you eat.

WHAT DO YOU EAT?

Fruit and vegetables are free (within reason) but everything else has a value, depending on which of their systems you are doing. A typical daily menu might be: **Breakfast:** Beans on Toast **Lunch:** Halloumi and Spinach with Beetroot **Dinner:** Homemade Fish and Chips. Recipes for these dishes can be found on pages 229–30.

WHAT IS BANNED?

Nothing is banned provided you keep track of the ProPoints value and are within your weekly and daily limits.

IS IT CHEAT FRIENDLY?

No. You get a number of ProPoints per week to use on treats, but everything has to be counted. That doesn't mean you can't spend your ProPoints on 'luxuries' like a beer or two.

WHAT MEN SAY
CRAIG MORRIS

Everything I love about Weight Watchers can be summed up in one word: spontaneity. I didn't get to nearly 19 stone by not being impetuous and since the idea behind most diets involves restrictions of one kind or another – be it no carbs, no dairy, no nitrogen or whatever – I like Weight Watchers' more open approach. Having a plan that allows me to eat whatever I fancy and easily understand how it affects the daily balance of my account is important to me.

The plan in its current incarnation allows followers to be spontaneous with their food choices by taking some fairly complex nutritional data into account and distilling it into an easy-to-understand numerical value. Thanks to tools like the app and calculator, it's a simple matter to work out the ProPoints value of any food you fancy on the fly (provided the nutritional info is available to you, which it often is). This makes Weight Watchers every bit as simple as calorie counting, without neglecting the simple fact that not all calories are created equal.

The science behind converting the protein, carbohydrate, fat and fibre of a Mars bar into a number makes me feel like I'm not making a bad choice when I grab one. More importantly, it works for me.

www.manvfat.com/members/craig-morris

THE MAN·FAT VIEW

One of the big draws of Weight Watchers is that, as with calorie counting, you can eat whatever you like. Fancy a doughnut? Have a doughnut! As long as you've got the points available, you can have whatever you like. Because of this it's really flexible and on some programmes the extra weekly bonus points allow you to go to restaurants, have a takeaway on a Friday night, or go for a pint with mates and still lose weight. An additional draw for some is the groups. Here you benefit from the support of a group and a 'leader' who is a first port of call for advice. You would need to decide whether the overwhelmingly female groups are something that would put you off, or possibly even be an attraction!

On the negative side you have to remember to measure and count everything. The only 'free' foods on Weight Watchers are fruit and most veg – everything else has to be counted, which can be pretty tedious. None of this comes free either and there is a monthly fee along with a joining fee. This gives you access to the mobile app, website and meetings, but this monthly fee will certainly add up if you've got a lot of weight to lose.

HOW TO GET STARTED

As one of the world's biggest weight-loss groups you should be able to find at least one Weight Watchers group near you – simply visit **www.manvfat.com/diets** and get more Weight Watchers information.

7 SLIMMING WORLD
Chosen by 4% of men

IN YOUR WORDS

- "I like the flexibility of Slimming World."
- "Slimming World is good because you never feel hungry."

HOW DO YOU DO IT?

With an emphasis on eating real food and a supportive meeting environment, Slimming World is a good choice if you love to cook from scratch, or if you want to learn how. Slimming World is one of the more complex diets to follow and the plan has changed in recent years; the current version has been christened the 'Extra Easy' plan, presumably by someone with a healthy grasp of irony. Here, one-third of every meal you have has to be 'Super Free' food (most fruits, vegetables and salad). The other two-thirds needs to be 'Free Foods' including lean meat, potatoes and pasta. The quantities of these free and superfree foods are not restricted.

You also have Healthy Extra choices to make during the day, which come in two forms. 'Healthy Extra A' is taken from your dairy food group, so for example, 320ml of skimmed milk, or 30g of cheese. 'Healthy Extra B' would be a fibre choice, equivalent to two slices of small wholemeal bread, or approximately 35g of cereals. Anything outside of these choices has a "Syn" value and you are allowed approximately 15 Syns per day when you first start the plan, although this does reduce as the weight comes off. These Syns can be used either on adding extras such as olive oil to your food, or you can use them for treats. Beer it is then which, depending on brand and size, can be anything up to 11.5 Syns.

WHAT DO YOU EAT?

A typical daily menu might look like: **Breakfast:** Take-away Yogurt and Granola Breakfast **Lunch:** Couscous Salad with Roasted Vegetables **Dinner:** Chicken and Pesto Pasta. Recipes for these dishes can be found on pages 230–2.

WHAT IS BANNED?

Slimming World is primarily a low-fat diet, so the sorts of foods that are restricted are those that are high in fat. Beyond this Syns are allowed which you can incorporate into your diet, based on the Syn values for different foods.

IS IT CHEAT FRIENDLY?

No, you need to fit any extras into your weekly Syn value.

WHAT MEN SAY
PHIL JONES

I've been doing Slimming World for two years. I've lost almost 147lbs (67kg) on the plan. It's fair to say that I've done every diet out there including Slimming World when it was red and green days. I lost weight with every plan whether it was Atkins, Slimfast or Weight Watchers, but always put it back on, usually with an extra stone. Doing that I yo-yoed between 27 and 24 stone for years.

With Slimming World it took me ages to get my head round the Healthy Extra choice thing. What I've learnt is that you really have to plan everything you intend to eat from first thing to last. This can cause all sorts of issues at first but I've found that writing a menu every three to four days and shopping for it has saved loads of food waste and stops me eating crap between meals and just throwing something together, which is usually rubbish food when I get in late from work.

The food you eat is what I call 'clean food' – whole ingredients and no processed foods – and if you like cooking and eating then this is the plan for you. It works best if you cook everything from scratch with fresh ingredients. I found the bread thing really hard as I had bread all day every day. I guess that is part of the reason I was the size I was! Slimming World doesn't really allow you to drink beer as it's loaded with Syns and trying to count them on a night out is virtually impossible. They do talk about 'Body Magic', or exercise as you and I would call it, but they don't really push this side of things.

The groups are very female-centred and I was the only bloke in our group for some time. I think because I have done so well it has helped to bring other guys to it. You only have to look at the magazine to see how female-focused it is. What I don't like is the sitting round listening to women go on as if it's confession time. They recommend you stay for the group sessions or 'IMAGE therapy' as they like to call it. To be honest the people that do well always stay. I have learnt some great tips about food and drink but I've also heard loads of people going on about this, that and the other far too often! As a bloke you tend to win the Slimmer of the Week award every week (as men often lose quicker than women) which upsets them a touch but hey ho! If you plan every meal, keep a food diary of everything you eat and stick to the plan you should lose about 3lb (1.3kg) a week most weeks until your body fat percentage gets much lower.

www.manvfat.com/members/philandfran

THE MAN v FAT VIEW

It is much harder to succeed on Slimming World if you don't know how to cook, so if you're looking to learn then Slimming World may be a good option. One bonus is that there's a massive list of unlimited foods. If you're hungry you can freely snack on eggs, ham and veggies and even if you fancy something sweet you can eat Müllerlight yogurts to your heart's content. Don't forget though that if you eat beyond your calorie limit you will find yourself struggling to lose weight.

There are supportive weekly meetings – again these are mostly women and again these are paid for. After being weighed at a Slimming World meeting, members take part in 'IMAGE therapy' (that stands for Individual Motivation and Group Experience) which helps to change your eating behaviour and it's good to see this area of weight loss being addressed. You can also ask questions and talk to the other members of your group during this time which can be handy when you need support.

You have to be organised to make Slimming World work for you and remember that you need to prepare your meals in advance. Perhaps the most annoying aspect of Slimming World is that it unnecessarily complicates food – you'll have to learn about Extra Easy days, Success Express days, Healthy Extras (but you'll get to know these as Hex A and Hex B), Free Foods, Superfree Foods, Speed Foods, Superspeed Foods as well as Syns and it can all be quite baffling. However, the biggest issue in my view is that it doesn't teach you much about portion control, which can potentially leave some damaging habits unaddressed.

HOW TO GET STARTED
Visit **www.manvfat.com/diets** to find your local Slimming
World group.

8 JUICE DETOX
Chosen by 3% of men

IN YOUR WORDS
- "I'm doing the Jason Vale detox programme."
- "Not all the time but I've started having a green juice for breakfast."
- "I've done a few juice fasts – not easy but a good kickstart."

HOW DO YOU DO IT?
Sometimes referred to as juice fasts, juice detoxes or simply detoxes, during a juice
detox you typically swap one or more meals for a vegetable and/or fruit juice.

As you might expect we're not talking cartons of shop-bought concentrated juice
here; this is more like a freshly squeezed kale, spinach and apple juice washed down
with a shot of wheatgrass. If it sounds extreme, that's because it is and real care
must be exercised to make sure that you are taking in enough calories to survive.

It's often touted as an easy way to lose weight with some programmes claiming that
you can lose 5lb (2.3kg) in just three days. There's often also some element of 'toxin
removal' promoted as part of the diet. The popularity of Joe Cross' documentary
Fat, Sick and Nearly Dead and 'Juice Master' Jason Vale's books have resulted
in many spin-offs and John Lewis has reported a 60% increase in sales of juice
machines since 2013.

WHAT DO YOU EAT?

A typical menu might include: **Breakfast:** Carrot, Apple and Ginger Juice **Lunch:**
Broccoli, Cucumber, Celery and Spinach Juice **Dinner:** Beetroot, Apple and Kale
Juice. Recipes for these juices can be found on page 233.

WHAT IS BANNED?

In many cases solid food is either banned or hugely restricted. Consequently,
anything you consume must be something that can be blended (no meat
smoothies, sadly).

IS IT CHEAT FRIENDLY?

No.

WHAT MEN SAY
DAN WOODWARD

After watching the documentary *Fat, Sick and Nearly Dead* I was inspired to
try and reboot my body with a juice fast. I loved how juicing made me feel,
the energy I had and the positive effects it had on my health and weight. I also
enjoyed a good deal of the recipes and how they re-tuned my taste buds. With
support from light exercise I lost 22lb (10kg) in my first four weeks of juicing,
and had never felt better in myself.

I didn't like running out of room in my fridge or cleaning the juicer! You may
also find some recipes not to your taste – especially ones with celery! I don't
like using the word detox: juicing is a reset of your body's systems; removing
synthetic stuff from the diet. In its place you supply your body with an
abundance of the raw building blocks of nutrition. Weight loss is often a side
effect of essentially experiencing calorie-controlled, healthy nutrition.

Juicing may seem like a thing you might find in an episode of *The Good Life*,

but I found it to be an effective way to prepare your body for a better lifestyle, or get back on track if you've lost your way.
www.manvfat.com/members/dan-woodward

THE MAN<small>v</small>FAT VIEW

There's no doubt that a switch to a juice detox plan feels like you're doing something serious about your weight. Although the concept of whether or not it actually works to detoxify the body is scientifically dubious, it certainly feels like it's purging you of something. Many of the juices are extremely tasty as well, although clearly that depends on your own preferences. The other obvious advantage is that you'll be getting lots of nutrients as every meal is packed full of fruit and veg. You can definitely achieve weight loss with juice detoxes. Cross lost 100lb (45kg) in 60 days drinking nothing but juice. That said, you also need to be aware that juices can be very high in calories, and that, separated from the pulp, the fruit and vegetables lose a lot of the fibre that makes them useful.

There are a lot of things to be aware of if you're going to do a juice plan. First, it's expensive – to make enough juice for a day you need a huge amount of fruit and veg, while the other expenditure is a juicer and they can be pricey. Also, switching to a liquid-only diet is tough. You will have spent decades equating food with chewing, and it often leaves you feeling a little hollow if all your consumption is simply slurped through a straw. Juice detoxes also need careful planning; going out during a detox is practically impossible, while if you're out at work you'll need to prepare your juices in advance.

The biggest note of caution is that juicing is, if anything, a short-term fix. If you're replacing one meal a day with a juice then that's different. Successful weight loss only counts if it's something you can sustain. There's very little point dropping 7lb (3kg) in a week, if the next week sees you return to your normal diet and put it back on again. And, as with all weight loss, you need to ensure that you are doing it safely – check your calorie consumption and if it falls under safe levels then seek medical advice before continuing.

HOW TO GET STARTED
Get a juicer, pick a programme to follow and start juicing. A good way into juicing is to find some recipes (see **www.manvfat.com/diets**) and try experimenting with them alongside whole food before deciding to replace entire meals with juices.

9 CAMBRIDGE DIET
Chosen by 2% of men

IN YOUR WORDS
- "I've looked at a number of Very Low Calorie Diets and I think the Cambridge one looks good."
- "I like the fact that you don't have to cook, you just buy the products and go."

HOW DO YOU DO IT?
The Cambridge Diet is a Very Low Calorie Diet (VLCD) where, under the guidance of a consultant, you eat Cambridge Diet meal-replacement products. There are six different programmes which range between 415 calories to 1,500 calories per day – the rate of your weight loss would depend on which you chose. You would either eat the meal-replacement products exclusively or in combination with normal foods. The products range from shakes, soups, porridges and bars. Over the course of your plan your calorie intake is gradually increased in stages which aim to bring you back to eating a varied and balanced diet by the end of the final stages.

WHAT DO YOU EAT?
A typical menu could consist of: **Breakfast:** Cambridge Diet Fruits of the Forest Shake **Lunch:** Cambridge Diet Leek and Potato Soup **Dinner:** Cambridge Diet Toffee and Walnut Shake **Snack:** Cambridge Lemon Yoghurt-Coated Bar.

WHAT IS BANNED?

Most non-Cambridge Diet foods until you progress past the first stage.

IS IT CHEAT FRIENDLY?

No.

WHAT MEN SAY
JON SALTER

I've done the Cambridge Diet four times over the course of about twenty years. I was attracted to it by the rapid weight loss and the simplicity of it – you have nothing to think about, everything is there for you and you know that all you can have is water, black coffee or tea and the four products per day. They do more products now like ready meals, but it's mostly a choice between the shakes, soups and bars.

There are five stages to the diet – the first is where you're just using the products and that's it. That can run from two weeks to much longer depending on how much you've got to lose. The most I've lost on it was 112lb (50.8kg) in six months. It can be tough at times, but it's incredibly quick weight loss. The problem I keep having is when you go to the next stages, like Stage Two where you have three Cambridge Diet products per day and green vegetables and white proteins like cottage cheese, eggs or chicken. You have to do that for a minimum of a week. You still lose weight at about three to four pounds per week.

During the first three days you feel really hungry and you do get the odd headache, but you can take paracetamol for that! After the third day you actually feel more alert and awake. You feel quite healthy. I'd say that if you're thinking of doing it then you should know that it's really good for quick weight loss but be careful on the progress to the next stages as that's where I keep slipping up.
www.manvfat.com/members/jon-salter-98

THE MAN‸FAT VIEW

Although it varies from person to person, many men have reported losing up to a stone a month while doing the Cambridge Diet, which can be very motivating. If you can stick to it without cheating, this diet plan should give you impressive results in a short space of time. Another advantage is that you don't have to think about preparing food. When trying to lose weight it can be difficult to figure out what exactly you should be eating and how much, but the good thing about the Cambridge Diet is that much of the time it's as complicated as opening one of their products. There's no weighing, counting, measuring or trying to navigate tricky-to-understand nutritional labels. Your Cambridge Diet Consultants are people who have personal experience of losing weight on the plan and they're there to support you by maintaining your personal records, answering any questions you have and cheering you on all the way.

Despite this there are many disadvantages to the plan, not least of which is the cost. It can make social situations difficult. Surviving on a liquid-only diet can feel quite socially isolating as you will be unable to join in with any food-related social activities. Aside from that you'll inevitably miss actual food. As with any VLCD you have to be aware that there will almost certainly be side effects. Dieters have reported headaches, tiredness, dizziness, nausea and diarrhoea. It's certainly not uncommon for men to lose weight on the Cambridge Diet and then regain it as soon as they stop doing it – perhaps suggesting that finding a more balanced plan to begin with would be advantageous for some men.

HOW TO GET STARTED
Visit **www.manvfat.com/diets** to find out more and get in touch with your local consultant.

10 SLOW CARB DIET/4-HOUR BODY
Chosen by 1% of men

IN YOUR WORDS

- "Slow carb from *The 4-Hour Body* book."
- "I'm doing The 4-Hour Body."
- "Any diet that gives me a day of cheating is OK by me."

HOW DO YOU DO IT?

Described as an 'Uncommon guide to rapid fat-loss, incredible sex and becoming superhuman', author Timothy Ferriss' book *The 4-Hour Body* outlines a diet plan for the time-poor modern man. Much more than just a diet, the book has tips to sort out every inch of your life – including how to sleep better and get better at sex.

The secret to losing weight the 4-Hour Body way is the 'Slow Carb' method, which is based on low-GI foods and follows just five rules:

- Avoid all white carbohydrates (bread, rice, pasta, etc)
- Don't eat fruit
- Cheat one day a week
- Don't drink calories
- Eat the same meals over and over

The diet also has a number of recommendations, such as eating 30g of protein within 30 minutes of waking up.

WHAT DO YOU EAT?

A lot of meat, lentils and vegetables. One possibly attractive quirk of the 4-Hour Body diet is that it allows for two glasses of red wine to be drunk per day. A typical daily menu might be: **Breakfast:** Omelette **Lunch:** Beef Stew **Dinner:** Prawn Stir-fry. Recipes for the above can be found on page 234–5.

WHAT IS BANNED?

Lots! Most of this is covered by the rules but primarily fruit and all simple (fast) carbohydrates.

IS IT CHEAT FRIENDLY?

Yes. One entire day per week is given aside to eating whatever you want.

WHAT MEN SAY
JASON BRINK

I chose 4HB because it made weight loss look easy and gave pretty simple and easy-to-follow steps for improvement. When I discovered it, I was in a very bad place and latched on to it like a life raft. I had tried so many other things, but not with enough willpower, and 4HB seemed like something I could do.

The eating schedule is easy and it can be followed relatively closely. You will not go hungry at all with 4HB... which is kind of a problem too. Sometimes, you need to go hungry and control your intake, not just cram yourself to the gills with 'slow burn carbs'. The diet has a large component of the 'eat as much as you want of these things', to it, and the reality is that you just really should not do that.

I would suggest if you're going to do this diet then you should track and control your intake. Just because it says you can eat all the beans you want does not mean you have free rein to sit on your couch eating bowls of chilli. You still need to get out there and exercise, and find a way to really track what you are eating.

www.manvfat.com/members/thatsitivehadit

THE MAN∨FAT VIEW

The 4-Hour Body is undoubtedly an interesting book that covers a huge range of weight and fitness topics and is well worth investigating. For the diet itself the main advantages are that you can eat whatever you like once a week and wine is built into your daily consumption! Ferriss says he goes out of his way to binge on ice cream and Snickers on Saturdays, going as far as to eat so much that he feels sick. By hugely restricting your simple carbohydrate intake it works in the same way as other low-carb high-fat plans and gives reliable weight loss.

That said, you will get bored. Ferriss recommends finding a few meals you enjoy and eating them ad nauseam – which depending on your view of lentils (one of the most commonly used sources of slow carbs) could get pretty nauseous, pretty quickly. Ferris states that this is a habit that the most successful dieters follow, but if you're a food lover and enjoy experiencing different cuisines, textures and flavours then this will feel restrictive. If you struggle with binge eating, this probably isn't the diet for you. The restrictions of the diet are countered by the weekly cheat day, where you can eat whatever you want – though this can be a slippery slope for some. Additionally, you need to make sure that your diet is within calorie restraints or you will find weight loss slow or impossible.

HOW TO GET STARTED

Pick up a copy of the book *The 4-Hour Body* and follow the rules it lays out. Check out **www.manvfat.com/diets** for more information and ideas.

GETTING ACTIVE

Remember the spoiler at the beginning of this Step that losing weight was about the magic ratio of 70% nutrition and 30% activity? Well, this is where that other 30% swings into action. And action really is the name of the game, because – unless you're struggling with basic concepts – 'activity' means you need to start moving more.

WHY ACTIVITY IS ESSENTIAL

Just to be clear – exercise is not essential for you to lose weight. You do not have to run, swim, jog, cycle, crunch, press or squat to burn fat. You can still create a calorie deficit if you do no form of activity or exercise whatsoever.

And yet, activity is essential. It may not be essential to weight loss but it is essential to life. Unless you are a statue, then movement is a basic function of being a human. Exercise is really just refining those movements so that you can get better at them. I've so far resisted the analogy of 'man as a machine' but I'm going to lapse for a second. If nutrition is the fuel that powers your body, then activity allows you to upgrade the individual components to improve the overall running of the machine.

TIP *Many diets allow you to eat more based on the activity that you do. You must be incredibly careful not to over-estimate the extra amount you can eat based on your activity. Many of the online estimates that are provided are wildly inaccurate and cannot factor in how hard you work during a session. Wrongly assuming you've 'earned' extra calories with exercise is a very common cause of the frustrating weight-loss plateaus. As a minimum, halve the number of calories your calculator says you've earned, or simply ignore it altogether and stick to your daily allowance, regardless of the extra you've earned. If you're training hard, just make sure you keep an eye on your overall calorie balance.*

BASIC MUSCLE GROUPS

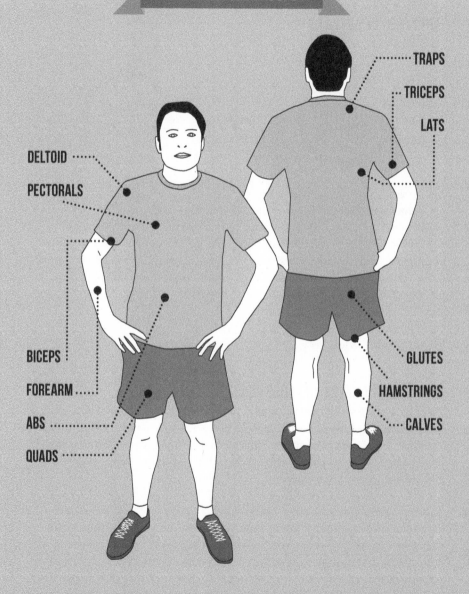

DELTOID

PECTORALS

BICEPS

FOREARM

ABS

QUADS

TRAPS

TRICEPS

LATS

GLUTES

HAMSTRINGS

CALVES

TWO TYPES OF ACTIVITY

There are two types of activity – the obligatory and the optional.

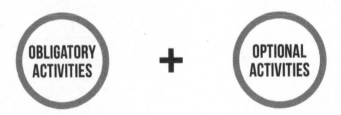

Are the things that you do in the course of a normal day that require movement or exertion. This may be things that you don't necessarily see as exercise, such as getting to work, moving around the house, errands (cleaning the house, picking up the children from school, etc). With smart thinking you can make these obligatory activities pay off in a big way for your weight loss.

Are what we would normally classify as exercise – the things that you choose to do over and above everyday life – playing sports or pursuing hobbies or the activities you do in an effort to get healthier, such as running or going to the gym.

WHY ACTIVITY HELPS YOU LOSE WEIGHT

There are two reasons why activity helps you lose weight. On the most basic level, activity forces the body to expend energy which can help to create a calorie deficit. The other way activity helps to lose weight is that it builds muscle. The muscle you build burns calories roughly three times faster than fat and you become a more efficient energy-burning machine.

Another important consideration is that muscle changes your body shape. If one of the reasons that you want to lose weight is because you want your appearance to change – to get rid of those man-boobs or that sagging gut – then activity is absolutely how you are going to do that. Your abdominal and back muscles are responsible for your core strength, but they are also what shapes your mid-section. Work on those muscles and, in combination with losing weight, you will start to see a radical change in the way that your gut looks. Same with your man-boobs. Develop your chest and pectoral muscles and, in combination with losing weight, you will start to see your shape change. Build arm and shoulder muscles and your body has a better sense of proportion, meaning you appear thinner.

REASONS NOT TO BE ACTIVE

When I started to exercise after losing a bit of weight I was terrified. I had a heart rhythm problem (partly as a result of being overweight) and even though several cardiologists had told me I was perfectly safe to exercise I'd built up a mental block with regard to activity.

I was terrified of it. I thought I'd die if I ran, either as a result of the sort of complete coronary explosion usually only seen in Tom and Jerry cartoons or simply from the shame of jiggling slightly more than your average jelly. Consequently, I chose all the most sedate pastimes and built up a mental picture of myself as someone who despised exercise. I thought people who went to the gym and went running were insane and annoying.

All of that thinking was to protect myself from the fear I felt about exercising. I started back with activity very slowly – and I mean incredibly slowly. What I quickly discovered is something that will come as no surprise to you – I don't hate activity at all, I love it. Activity brings purpose, it feeds your motivation. It provides you with many exciting and fulfilling challenges. It's a fantastic social occasion. It blows away the cobwebs. It lifts depression. It gives you energy. In short, I have now become one of those people I used to think was insane and annoying. Join us!

Interestingly, fear didn't feature in the reasons revealed by the Big Fat Survey as to why men say they are not more active. Despite that, you can probably see from the answers that the root of a lot of these reasons for missing out is simply fear by a different name.

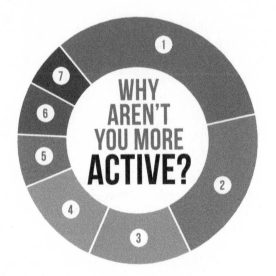

1. **NO TIME, MONEY OR ENERGY**
   33%
2. **FEEL EMBARRASSED**
   21%
3. **INJURY, ILLNESS OR DISABILITY**
   14%
4. **CAN'T BE BOTHERED**
   12%
5. **NO IDEA HOW TO START**
   7%
6. **WORRIED ABOUT HEALTH**
   7%
7. **HATE ALL SPORTS**
   6%

1. NO TIME, MONEY OR ENERGY

Chosen by 33% of men

This translates as – 'I don't value myself enough to make activity enough of a priority'. You can resist that statement as much as you want. You can throw this book down and curse the name of MAN v FAT, but this is a statement that needs challenging. If you are saying that you don't exercise because of time, money, energy, or you simply 'can't be bothered' then you are living off excuses. If during the course of a normal day you move (whether it's to work, around the house, whatever) then you already have the capability to use your obligatory activity to get fitter for free.

Claiming that you don't have enough energy to exercise may be attached to a deeper fear, possibly related to self-esteem or depression. If so, this is something that should be dealt with properly – see Step One (page 36). For most, though, it is simply an excuse which overlooks some fundamental truths about exercise. Yes, there is a phase while you exercise during which your muscles get fatigued, you breathe hard and you sweat. When that phase is over though the body is swamped by a feeling of euphoria similar to the feeling you experience after sex. Combine this with your body's enhanced ability to process oxygen and activity is a guaranteed way of actually *creating*, not losing, energy.

2. FEEL EMBARRASSED
Chosen by 21% of men

For many men this is the key. We have been inactive for so long that it's flat-out embarrassing to consider signing up for a gym, or going for a run. What would the neighbours say? If switching off the part of your brain that cares what other people think isn't an option, then consider the different forms of activity – obligatory and optional. Start very slowly on improving your obligatory activity – no one need ever know that you are getting fit (there's never a need for skin-tight neon lycra). You can also do many optional activities in your own home. A DVD or a simple bodyweight programme can be all you need to get fit without embarrassment (see Fitness Plans on pages 112–33 and **www.manvfat.com/resources**).

3. INJURY, ILLNESS OR DISABILITY
Chosen by 14% of men

Injuries are often caused by people who are not used to activity suddenly getting back into it without taking the proper steps. If you start by doing a tiny amount and build it up very slowly, then you hugely minimise your risk of injury. Citing an injury, illness or disability is still an excuse, though. There are very few conditions that prevent all movement and, unless you're in an iron lung, you can find ways to improve your levels of movement. If you can't think of a way around your injury, illness or disability – or you're simply worried about your health and how safe it is to start getting active – then raise the situation with your doctor. They should have plenty of suggestions about how to progress. If they don't, then get a better doctor.

4. CAN'T BE BOTHERED
Chosen by 12% of men

See no time, money or energy.

5. NO IDEA HOW TO START
Chosen by 7% of men

Then you're in the right place! Read on for all of the information and guidance you need to help improve your activity levels and fitness with both obligatory and optional exercise.

6. WORRIED ABOUT HEALTH
Chosen by 7% of men

See injury, illness or disability.

7. HATE ALL SPORTS
Chosen by 6% of men

This is a great cheat. In your mind you've built up a picture of yourself as someone who prefers to sit and watch television or play computer games, rather than be outside doing exercise. You might have a poor relationship with sports from school where you hated P.E. lessons or perhaps you just hate sports as a whole and find the time other men spend on football, cricket or baseball a complete mystery. That's fine – you're the guy who doesn't like sports. That doesn't mean that you have to write off all activity, though. As we'll see, activity has a far wider scope than simply chasing balls of various shapes around a field.

OBLIGATORY ACTIVITY

Learning how to increase your obligatory activity is very simply a case of doing an audit of all the movement you need to do in the course of a day and making smarter choices with regard to how you do them. If you'd normally pick the children up in the car, then swap it for walking to school. It doesn't have to be every day – start with once a week and plan to increase it where possible. If you usually drive to work, figure out a way to swap this for a bike or a walking commute. Or get off the train or bus a stop early and build up from there. Improving your obligatory activity is a game that we should all play – right now, start examining your life and find ways that you can enjoyably improve your activity levels.

START SMALL

Don't suddenly sell your car and insist on walking everywhere – do a survey of your life and identify 10 points where you can move more. Start thinking about how and when you can introduce those improvements.

Here are some ideas:
- Do you take phone calls sitting down?
- How do you get to work?
- Where and when do you walk?
- Can you get a pedometer or an activity watch? (See page 174 for more on this.)
- List the errands you do on a weekly basis – how can you make them burn more calories?
- What journeys do you do on a weekly basis?
- What is your working situation like?
- Could you switch to a standing desk?
- What do you do in the evenings?
- Can you choose to carry some extra weight in your bag – a sheaf of paper or a litre water bottle?
- How often do you use the lift or escalator?
- When you socialise, can you trade up what you do, or the way you get there?

Not all of these points will be relevant to you, but some will and your challenge is to capitalise on these to produce a list of things that you can gradually introduce into your life in the coming weeks. Don't make the mistake of thinking that these sort of little things don't make a massive difference. Small changes plus time will equal a huge difference.

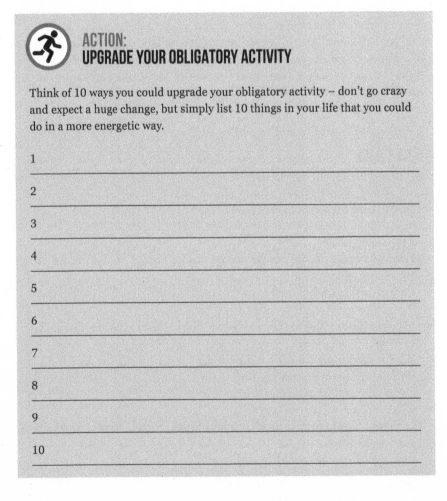

ACTION:
UPGRADE YOUR OBLIGATORY ACTIVITY

Think of 10 ways you could upgrade your obligatory activity – don't go crazy and expect a huge change, but simply list 10 things in your life that you could do in a more energetic way.

1

2

3

4

5

6

7

8

9

10

OPTIONAL ACTIVITY

The single biggest mistake that men make when it comes to optional activity is that they elect to do things that they hate. It's actually baffling. Often this happens because they get some advice from a well-meaning friend who gives them a brutal gym plan or perhaps, in a moment of weakness, they believe the promises and buy the Abdominator 4000. However it happens, the result is that you start an optional activity plan you hate. Perhaps you can grit your teeth and complete the programme – very few will – but every single day you're doing it you will hate it and want it to be over. In time this will colour your experience of exercise and cheat you of the elation of finding optional activities you love.

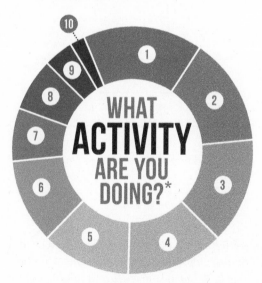

WHAT ACTIVITY ARE YOU DOING?*

*OR THINKING ABOUT DOING?

1. **WALKING** 16%
2. **RUNNING** 14%
3. **SWIMMING** 14%
4. **CYCLING** 13%
5. **GOING TO THE GYM** 12%
6. **WEIGHTLIFTING** 11%
7. **FITNESS CLASSES** 7%
8. **YOGA** 7%
9. **RUGBY** 4%
10. **FOOTBALL** 2%

There is an alternative – finding something active that you actually love doing, then progressively doing more of it. It really doesn't matter what activity it is. If you love it and it makes you more flexible, fitter or stronger – do more of it. So what actually counts as an activity? Bottom line: anything that requires movement or exercise counts as an activity. Walking, running, jumping, swimming, cycling. For comparison the activities listed on the previous page are the optional activities that the Big Fat Survey showed most men were interested in getting into.

If you're looking to start then pick one of our Fitness Plans which can help you to slowly and safely get back into these optional activities, many of them without even leaving your house. Right now, commit to finding optional activities you love – there are free taster sessions of pretty much any activity you care to mention and with just a switch of your mental approach you can be out there finding one that really does it for you:

I'm going to try:

1
_____

2
_____

3
_____

4
_____

5
_____

TIP *Not all optional activities are equal when it comes to weight loss. If you're looking at optional activity as something that you want to do purely to burn calories then it might help to pick a sport that burns them quickly. Bear in mind the figures opposite are very approximate because the amount of energy you burn will be dependent on your own situation – primarily your weight – but they can be useful as a comparison.*

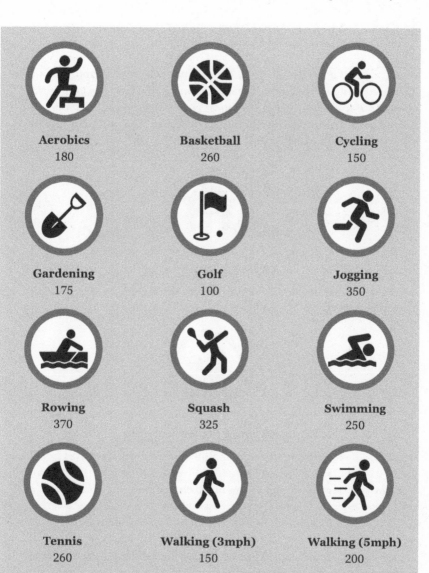

Aerobics
180

Basketball
260

Cycling
150

Gardening
175

Golf
100

Jogging
350

Rowing
370

Squash
325

Swimming
250

Tennis
260

Walking (3mph)
150

Walking (5mph)
200

Calories expended over 30 minutes of exercise, all values approximate.

MAKING YOUR FITNESS PLANS

Don't panic if you're looking at the various optional activities that are out there and feel that they're just too much of a leap for you at the moment. For example, if you'd enjoy going to the gym but worry that people would laugh at you then there is hope. Two of the best ways of getting back into exercise are:

STARTING SLOWLY AT HOME

It's very common to build your way up to being able to go to the gym with some simple home exercises.

WORK WITH A PERSONAL TRAINER

If you have some money to spend on your fitness then investing in a personal trainer can be a brilliant idea as you will get personalised and appropriate exercise to help you achieve your goals. You also know that there is a safety net of someone looking out for you as you exercise – even a few sessions can be enough to set a very gentle plan and build the confidence needed to start putting it into action.

If you're working out alone it can be useful to understand how hard you're working so that you can keep an eye on whether you're progressing or not – for this you can either use a heart rate monitor, or if you'd prefer something simpler and cheaper then the talk test is often just as effective.

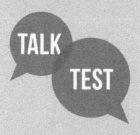

TALK TEST

The Talk Test is a simple way to judge how hard you are pushing yourself.

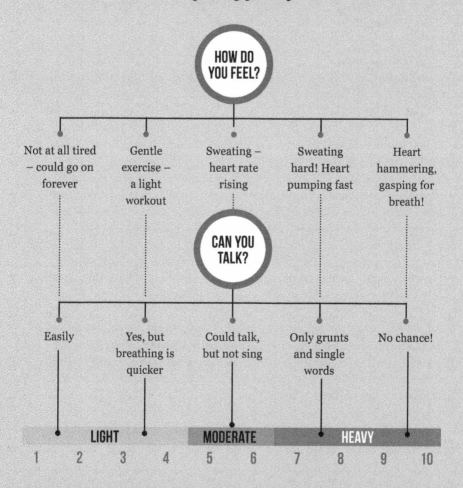

HOW DO YOU FEEL?

Not at all tired – could go on forever

Gentle exercise – a light workout

Sweating – heart rate rising

Sweating hard! Heart pumping fast

Heart hammering, gasping for breath!

CAN YOU TALK?

Easily

Yes, but breathing is quicker

Could talk, but not sing

Only grunts and single words

No chance!

LIGHT   MODERATE   HEAVY

1   2   3   4   5   6   7   8   9   10

You can broadly split fitness into three types – all of which should be accounted for in your optional activity plans.

Cardiovascular
The stuff that works your heart, makes you sweat and breathe hard.

Flexibility
The stuff that makes you stretch and bend.

Strength
The stuff that makes you sweat, breathe hard, stretch, bend and builds muscle.

Any plan which doesn't consider each of these elements is not balanced and will be more likely to lead to injuries. Don't be the guy who can bench press two times his body weight but can't run to catch a bus. Regardless of your overall fitness goals, a balance of these disciplines will give you the most well-rounded approach.

You will notice that all of these Fitness Plans are incredibly slow; that's because there's absolutely no harm in taking things really slow to start with. The aim here is to get back into these activities, not to become a master, just yet.

After the initial 30-day period you should find that your abilities have improved, it should have impacted on your weight and also how you feel about trying out exercise again. At this point you can consider going further and getting involved with organised activities, or simply starting the programme again but increasing the distance, weight or effort.

Before you begin you should consider making an appointment with your doctor to confirm that you are healthy enough to exercise.

WALKING FITNESS PLAN

Perfect for anyone looking for a slow introduction back into running, or wanting to find ways to make walking more effective at burning fat. If a phase is too easy, skip to the next one.

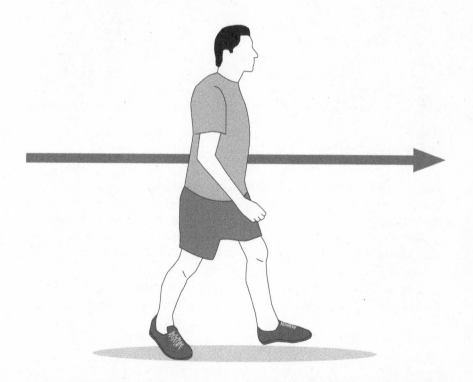

TIP *During any 30-day plan you will have good days and bad days. The important thing is to keep focus and stick with the plan. We all have off days but don't give up and try to get back on track as soon as you can.*

PHASE ONE **MARCHING**

Days 1–5

On Day 1, march on the spot for 20 steps. Increase the steps by 10 per day so that on Day 5 you will march 60 steps in total.

Day 6 Rest.

 If you cannot manage 20 steps on Day 1 don't worry – do what you can and make a note of how many steps you did. Every day try to do more than the day before.

PHASE TWO **VERTICAL**

Days 7–11

Start by standing on the floor in front of the bottom step of a staircase or any step of a similar height (approx. 180mm). Step your right foot up onto the stair followed by the left. Once both feet are on the stair, step your right foot back down, followed by the left. Do this 10 times. Repeat, leading with the left foot 10 times. This will give you a complete set of 20 step-ups.

Each day increase your set by 2 step-ups. On Day 8 you will do 11 with the right then 11 with the left. Day 9, 12 with the right, 12 with the left, and so on.

Day 12 Rest.

PHASE THREE **DISTANCE**

Days 13–17

Get your trainers, grab a watch, get outside and start walking. On Day 13 walk for 2 minutes then turn around and go back to your start point. This will mean a total of 4 minutes walking. Make a note of where you got to and write it down. Every day increase your outbound time by 15 seconds (this will increase your total walk time by 30 seconds). On Day 17 you will be walking non-stop for 6 minutes.

To see how far you've progressed, on Day 17 make a note of how long it takes you to get to the point you noted on Day 13.

Day 18 Rest.

PHASE FOUR INTERVALS

Days 19–23

Once again, these walks will be done outside. On Day 19 start with 5 minutes walking. Take a 2-minute rest before returning to your starting point. Increase your walk time by 1 minute and decrease your rest time by 10 seconds every day. By Day 23 you should be walking for nine minutes, resting for 1 minute 20 seconds one way, then walking back to your starting point for nine minutes.

Day 24 Rest.

PHASE FIVE ACTIVE INTERVALS

Days 25–29

Day 25 – start with a 10-minute walk. During this walk go at a normal pace for 50 steps then increase the pace as much as you can comfortably for 10 steps then revert to normal pace for 50 steps. Repeat these intervals of higher effort for the entire 10-minute set.

Increase the work each day by adding 2 minutes to the length of your walk. So on Day 26 you would walk for 12 minutes, while by Day 29 you should be walking for 18 minutes with the intervals described above.

Day 30 Rest and choose your next plan!

 TIP *For a further progression walk 50 steps/ fast walk 10 steps/ light jog 10 steps and increase as above.*

RUNNING FITNESS PLAN

This is a good, slow plan to introduce you to running. Before embarking on this plan you should have completed the 30-day walking fitness plan and be able to walk comfortably for 20 minutes. You don't want to run before you can... you get the point. Remember to work on your flexibility to reduce the chance of injuries. It's also vital that you have good-quality trainers, a watch (or smartphone) and somewhere to record your times.

PHASE ONE STAMINA

Days 1–5
On Day 1, complete a 20-minute steady-paced walk. Increase this by 5 minutes every day. By Day 5 your steady walk should last for 40 minutes.

Day 6 Rest.

 TIP *This might seem like a big daily increase but remember you are walking only at this point, building up your stamina and endurance.*

PHASE TWO INTERVALS

Days 7–11
On day 7, go for a 20-minute walk. Start at a steady pace for 5 minutes then jog for 10 steps. Walk a further 5 minutes then jog again for 10 steps. Continue this for a 20-minute session with 4 intervals of 10 jogging steps.

Work for 20 minutes every day in this phase adding in more jogging intervals of 10 steps. On Day 8 jog every 4 minutes. On Day 9 jog every 3 minutes. On Day 10 jog every 2 minutes and on Day 11 jog 10 steps every 1 minute.

Day 12 Rest.

PHASE THREE LONGER SESSION

Days 13–17

On Day 13, complete a 20-minute walk with 10 jogging steps every minute. Keeping the same jogging step intervals of 10 steps every minute of walking, increase the time of your session by 2 minutes every day, so that on Day 17 you will be doing a 28-minute session with 28 jogging step intervals.

Day 18 Rest.

PHASE FOUR PROGRESSION

Days 19–23

On Day 19 revert to a 20-minute session, but increase the number of jogging steps per minute to 15. Increase the number of jogging steps per minute by 5 steps each day so that on day 20 you will walk for a minute and jog for 20 steps every minute, while by day 23 you will be walking for a minute then jogging for 35 steps.

Day 24 Rest.

PHASE FIVE RUNNING MAN!

Days 25–30

DAY 25 – Set your clock for 5 minutes, walk for 1 minute then jog for as long as you can up to 5 minutes (1 minute walk, 4 minutes jog). Repeat this for a session of 20 minutes with four 1-minute periods of walking. Once you can jog for the full 4 minutes then reduce your walking time by 30 seconds. Keep going until you can run for the full 20 minutes. Then look to increase this to 30 by adding 2 minutes to your session time.

Day 31 Rest and choose your next plan!

If you cannot jog for the full 4 minutes then repeat for the 6 days until you can, trying to increase the jog time each session.

BODYWEIGHT STRENGTH FITNESS PLAN

A perfect challenge if you want to build strength away from a gym. For this all you need is a bit of floor space and a wall. You are going to be looking at THREE key exercises. These can be built upon as you gain strength through the movements and, of course, lose weight.

The exercises are: the Push-up, the Squat and the Bridge. Over the next 30 days we are going to work these three exercises in a structured system following a weekly template of the number of times you complete each exercise (these are called repetitions, or reps) and the number of times you complete these reps (these are called sets).

Each week you will complete the following number of reps and sets of the three exercises for 6 days, then rest on day 7. For each of these take 1 minute's rest between sets.

- **Week 1** – 3 reps x 5 sets
- **Week 2** – 4 reps x 4 sets
- **Week 3** – 5 reps x 4 sets
- **Week 4** – 8 reps x 3 sets

For example a set in Week 1 would consist of 3 push-ups, 3 squats and 3 bridges followed by a 1-minute rest, while a set in Week 4 would consist of 8 push-ups, 8 squats and 8 bridges.

THE EXERCISES

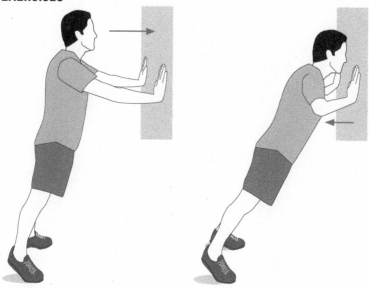

THE PUSH-UP

1. Stand facing a wall, with the palms of your hands on the wall at your shoulder height and width.

2. Slowly lower your forehead to the wall, pause for a second then push back through your arms to the start position. Remember to keep your stomach tight and try to lock your body so that it is like a plank of wood with just your arms performing the movement.

 Make it tougher: *Move your feet further away from the wall. If this is still too easy do your push-up on the floor, either with knees dropped to the floor or in a classic push-up pose.*

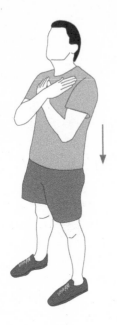

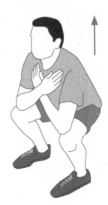

THE SQUAT

1. Stand upright with your feet slightly wider than shoulder-width apart, your arms crossed across your chest and with your toes pointing forward.

2. Looking up at the ceiling and pushing your chest forward as you move, slowly bend your knees and push your bum backwards, as if you're sitting down onto an imaginary chair. Go as low as you feel comfortable with at first and try not to bend forward as you go. Pause for a second and then push through your heels to return to the starting position.

 Make it tougher: *Bend your knees more with each squat to increase the depth of the movement.*

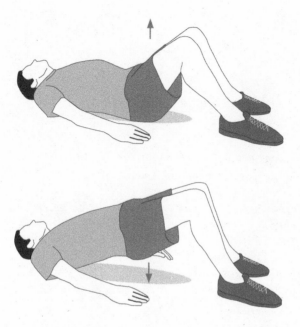

THE BRIDGE

1. Lie on your back on the floor with your knees bent and your feet flat and as close to your bum as you can get them. Place your hands on the floor by your sides, palms facing down, and tuck your chin forward into your chest. This is your start position.

2. From this position push through your heels and hands and try to lift your bum off the ground. If you can, pause for a second before lowering slowly back down. If you can't, then just hold the tension through your body for a second before lowering yourself back into the starting position.

Make it tougher: *Place your hands on the opposite shoulders (by crossing your arms) and push up through the heels only.*

TROUBLESHOOTING

TIMING

On all of the exercises work to a 1-1-1 tempo. One second into the exercise, one second pause, one second out of the exercise.

CAN'T DO THE REPS?

If you cannot manage the full amount of reps simply make a note of what you can do and try to add a rep in every day.

REST TIME

Try to stick to 1 minute between sets, however if this isn't long enough extend your rest time but try not to rest for longer than 2 minutes.

WEIGHT TRAINING FITNESS PLAN

If you're interested in getting into weight training then this plan will give you an introduction to some of the key exercises and start to build your strength. It's advisable to follow the bodyweight strength fitness plan before progressing onto the external loading (weight training) sets here, however it is not essential that you do so.

Equipment required – two dumbbells or kettlebells of equal weight. Don't go too heavy on these as we're looking at perfecting the technique and getting you used to the lifting process. For these initial sets of exercises these should be no heavier than 5kg (11lb) per weight. Eventually you need to be lifting a lot heavier to build your strength, but for now let's get the movements done properly.

The exercises are: the Shoulder Press, the Bent-over Row and the Deadlift.

As with the bodyweight strength fitness plan, we are going to break these workouts into weekly sets, working 6 days and resting on the seventh. Likewise, once again we are going to structure the reps and sets as with the bodyweight plan. We will be working towards 3 sets of 8 repetitions. Once you have mastered the exercise form and can complete this number of movements with ease, simply increase the weight and work your way back up to 3 sets of 8 repetitions. For each take 1 minute's rest between sets.

So the structure of the plan is going to look like this:

- **Week 1** – 3 reps x 5 sets
- **Week 2** – 4 reps x 4 sets
- **Week 3** – 5 reps x 4 sets
- **Week 4** – 8 reps x 3 sets

For example, a set in Week 1 would consist of 3 deadlifts, 3 shoulder presses and 3 bent-over rows followed by a 1-minute rest, while a set in Week 4 would consist of 8 deadlifts, 8 shoulder presses and 8 bent-over rows.

THE EXERCISES

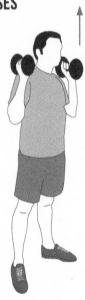
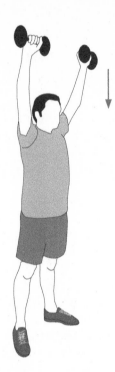

THE SHOULDER PRESS

The shoulder press is another multi-muscle move that is going to work the pushing muscles of the arms, chest and shoulders. We are going to work this exercise while standing up and therefore engaging the core and abdominal muscles at the same time. This approach will eventually make all of your workouts more economical.

1. Grab your weights and stand upright. Bring the weights up level with your shoulders with your thumbs pointing behind you and elbows tucked in to your sides. This is your start position.

2. Drive the weights upwards in a smooth motion, tracking the elbows all the way through the movement, making sure that they don't flare out to the sides. Pause at the top then bring the weights back down in a slow, controlled manner back to the start position. This counts as one rep.

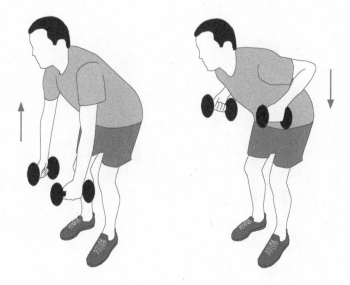

THE BENT-OVER ROW

The bent-over row will work the major pulling muscles of the arms and back and, as with the shoulder press, it's going to be performed standing up, so that the core and abdominal muscles get a workout too.

1. Stand upright holding the weights by your sides and level with your hips, with your thumbs pointing forward. Bending at the hips, lean forward as far as is comfortable, keeping the head high. Roll your shoulders back and try to get the shoulder blades to touch; this will extend your chest forwards. Bend your knees slightly and look up towards the ceiling. This is your start position (also known as the gorilla posture).

2. Pull the weights as high upwards into your armpits as you can, then pause for a second before lowering them back to the start position. This counts as one rep. Remember to stay in the gorilla posture for the whole of your set.

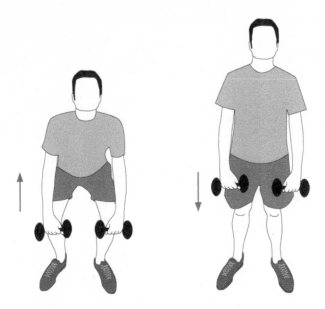

THE DEADLIFT

The deadlift is known as the 'king of all lifts' and rightly so. It is a huge compound move that recruits most of the major muscle groups in the body. It is a strongman staple and it is a common aim to want to deadlift two to three times your own bodyweight. For us, though, just the mechanics of the deadlift motion can increase mobility, flexibility, motor skills and strength, even with a relatively light weight.

1. Stand upright with your feet shoulder-width apart. Set your dumbbells or kettlebells on the floor about 6 inches (15cm) to the side of each heel.

2. Using the squat movement from the bodyweight set, bend your knees and take your bum backwards whilst keeping your head high and back straight. Let your arms hang by your sides as you squat. Keep looking forward and take hold of the weights when you reach the low point of your squat. Roll your shoulders back and try to pinch your shoulder blades together.

3. Grab hold of the weights and reverse the squat motion, ensuring that the chest is pushed forward and the head is high throughout the upwards movement. Push your hips forward as if somebody is pulling you by the belt buckle as you drive up. At the top of the move you should be back to standing upright again but this time with the weights in your hands. To complete the deadlift, repeat the whole movement but this time when you get to the bottom of the squat gently place the weights back on to the floor before performing the second part of the movement. Once the weights are on the floor and you are back in the starting position you have completed one rep.

TROUBLESHOOTING

TIMING

On all of the exercises work to a 1-1-1 tempo. One second into the exercise, one second pause, one second out of the exercise.

BREATHING

Breathing is very important, especially when you start lifting heavier weights. Always breathe out on the exertion (the hardest part) of any exercise. For the three exercises described here you should breathe out AS THE WEIGHTS GO UP i.e. on the upwards part of all of the exercises. Just remember the breathing OUT part, the breathing in will take care of itself.

CAN'T DO THE REPS?

If you cannot manage the full amount of reps simply make a note of what you can do and try to add a rep in every day.

REST TIME

Try to stick to 1 minute's rest between sets. If, however, you feel this isn't long enough you can extend your rest time, but try not to rest for any longer than 2 minutes.

CYCLING FITNESS PLAN

This plan is ideal if you would like to get up to cycling for an hour per session, which would not only burn approximately 300 calories, but would also open up the possibility of commuting by bike and the possibility of looking for cycling events and clubs to join.

The plan is tough but achievable, there are lots of rest days built in and it is recommended that you use them for stretching, reading and researching. You shouldn't need any special foods or products to support you on this plan, just a bike, a pair of padded cycling shorts, a helmet, plenty of good healthy meals and water.

Cycling, like running, is a 'narrow' sport so consequently you need to open up the body. This is where swimming and yoga or stretching come in. At a minimum it is vital to stretch out gently after each session, even for five minutes. Failure to do this can result in injuries.

 If you haven't ridden for a long time, get your bike serviced and ensure that it's set up correctly, paying particular attention to the height of the saddle and handlebars. Check your bike before every ride.

 Too tough?
If you are finding this programme too difficult then simply divide all the sessions in half and progress to doing this plan the following month.

	WEEK 1	WEEK 2	WEEK 3	WEEK 4
Monday	20 minute gentle cycle	30 minute gentle ride	30 minute ride	Hill reps* x 7
Tuesday	REST	REST	REST	REST
Wednesday	REST	Hill reps* x3	Hill reps* x 5	50 minute ride
Thursday	REST	REST	REST	REST
Friday	30 minute ride	30 minute ride	45 minute ride as fast as you can safely	REST
Saturday	REST	REST	REST	REST
Sunday	30 minute ride	40 minute ride as fast as you can safely	45-60 minute ride	60 minute ride as fast as you can safely

*HILL REPS

During this exercise find a nearby hill. Time yourself cycling up the hill from bottom to top. As you repeat, try to make sure that your time is the same or better, even when it's the last rep. This should be challenging, but it's the best way to build strength and stamina.

SWIMMING FITNESS PLAN

For this plan – which gets you back into a good swimming weight-loss routine – you will need to swim three times per week. Many pools open early and have adult and lane sessions in the evening as well as at lunch time. Make the most of these opportunities and on rest days make sure you are working on your strength and flexibility – both of which will improve your performance in the pool.

During these swims you can use any stroke you feel comfortable with, but as you progress record the number of lengths you do on front crawl and try and improve this at each session, with the aim to do 100% of your lengths using front crawl in the future. If you need to rest, take very short but frequent breaks – for example, take a 10 second rest every 5 minutes. Ideally, learn to rest by simply switching to a less demanding stroke for a couple of lengths.

You will need: trunks, comfortable goggles, earplugs, a water bottle and a pull buoy or float.

TIP
A reasonable goal for progression in this month-long plan is to aim to be able to swim a mile by the end of the programme. A mile in a 25-metre pool will be 64 lengths or 32 lengths in a 50-metre pool. Don't worry if you don't reach this level – being able to swim for 40 minutes will be great for cardio and strength.

	WEEK 1	WEEK 2	WEEK 3	WEEK 4
Monday	15 minute swim	20 minute swim – use the float to swim legs only for at least 5 minutes	25 minute swim – use the float to swim legs only for at least 6.5 minutes	30 minute swim – use the float to swim legs only for at least 7.5 minutes
Tuesday	**REST**	**REST**	**REST**	**REST**
Wednesday	15 minute swim – use the pull buoy for 3 minutes of the session to work the upper body	20 minute swim – use the pull buoy for 5 minutes of the session to work the upper body	25 minute swim – use the pull buoy for 6.5 minutes of the session to work the upper body	30 minute swim – use the pull buoy for 7.5 minutes of the session to work the upper body
Thursday	**REST**	**REST**	**REST**	**REST**
Friday	**REST**	**REST**	**REST**	**REST**
Saturday	20 minute swim – aim to swim as far as you can in this session and keep a note of the number of lengths	25 minute swim – aim to swim as far as you can in this session and keep a note of the number of lengths	30 minute swim – aim to swim as far as you can in this session and keep a note of the number of lengths	40 minute swim – aim to swim as far as you can in this session and keep a note of the number of lengths
Sunday	**REST**	**REST**	**REST**	**REST**

GOOD HABITS TO MAKE, BAD HABITS TO BREAK

Regardless of which diet you are choosing to follow there will be other factors at play that can impact on your weight. These are the good habits that will improve your fat loss and make you healthier, and the bad habits you should look to eliminate.

- Sleeping
- Clean eating
- Cheating
- Mindful eating
- Hydration
- Intermittent fasting
- Probiotics and prebiotics
- Meditation and breathing techniques

SLEEPING

There's every chance you're not getting enough shut-eye. One third of men do not get enough sleep – with the magic number of Zs resting between seven and eight hours of slumber. Why is poor sleep bad for your weight loss? Consider the study that found if you sleep for less than five hours per night then you are 33% more likely to gain 30 pounds than someone who slept for seven hours a night. So what's your sleeping pattern like – do you get enough? Take the Health Report at **www. manvfat.com/healthreport** to see.

There are some startling reasons why too little sleep impacts on your weight loss. For a start, because you're tired your body starts to crave more energy-dense foods, hoping to swiftly boost your flagging energy levels. Of course, you can fight those feelings but that's a willpower battle that you simply do not need to fight.

Feeling tired is also a key reason for skipping exercise and opting for easier obligatory activity – jumping in the car rather than walking, for example. Additionally, your body slows down your metabolism when it's tired – which of course has a huge impact on how quickly you're losing weight. Finally, the less you sleep, the higher your cortisol levels.

Like most healthy habits, getting enough sleep is simply a case of having a plan, sticking to it and refining it. Follow these tips and monitor your sleep to ensure you're getting enough quality slumber.

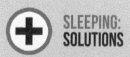

SLEEPING:
SOLUTIONS

- *Make sure your bedroom is set up for great sleep – the curtains should exclude all light and it should be as quiet as possible – alternatively consider an eye-mask and ear-plugs.*
- *Your mattress, sheets, duvet and pillows should be clean and comfortable.*
- *Get rid of phones and all light or noise sources as much as possible. Buy an alarm clock rather than using your mobile.*
- *Switch off all electronic devices at least an hour before bed.*
- *Try meditation before you sleep to calm your mind.*
- *If you find it hard to switch off, make a list of the things that are in your head and promise yourself you'll attend to the list in the morning.*
- *Experiment with camomile, valerian root tea and warm milky drinks.*
- *Only look at sleeping pills as a very last resort.*

CLEAN EATING

In essence, clean eating is a move towards rejecting processed and refined foods and focusing instead primarily on fresh, whole foods. Another angle to clean eating is that it looks to promote foods that are environmentally friendly – with a preference for organic fruits and vegetables, and meat and fish from organic and cruelty free environments.

This is important for several reasons, but primarily because of what is lost and gained when food is processed. Processed food often includes chemical additives because the food needs to survive for longer than it normally would. A source of huge concern are the sugars and trans fatss that food manufacturers manage to squeeze into many of their products. Equally, as soon as food is picked and processed it starts to lose the nutrients that make it biologically useful. In short, you end up eating something that seems like food, but is actually a pale imitation – or rather it would be a pale imitation if it hadn't been primped and fluffed with colourings.

If you're interested in moving towards clean eating then the simplest way of doing it is to apply the great-grandmother test to everything you eat. If an ancient relative would have recognised what you are eating as food then it's fine – if she wouldn't then you should dump it. Stick to food without packaging – buy avocados rather than shop-bought guacamole.

CHEATING

Many of us have spent years cheating on diets and often our weekly eating is more cheat days than diet days. If you've not come across the term before it simply means a period of time – usually either a single meal or an entire day – where you suspend your normal rules, often dramatically.

Some diets like 5:2 and the 4-Hour Body (see pages 77 and 97) are built and sold on the concept of the cheat day and often cheating crops up among more restrictive diets, where without a release valve you might struggle to stay on the diet. On other diets like Weight Watchers and Slimming World the 'cheats' are built into your daily allowance and sometimes you can save these up for one big splurge per week.

There are two prime reasons that people put forward for cheating:
- A psychological boost
- To 'kick-start' your metabolism

The psychological boost comes when you consider that following a diet that significantly cuts down on what you can eat can be really tough. There's nothing to make you want a slice of toasted white bread more than someone saying that it's explicitly forbidden. If, however, you can defer the things you are 'robbed of' to your cheat day/meal then it gets significantly easier to withstand the temptations.

The metabolism issue is harder to determine. The theory is that as you follow a weight-loss programme your body slows the metabolic function down to cope with the lower incoming calorie load. With the sudden intake of calories that goes with a cheat day/meal this 'tricks' the body into speeding up the metabolism again and allows your weight-loss rate to continue.

I've personally found cheat meals work for me, but I try to follow them in a balance now because there are some significant dangers with cheating:
- It requires real willpower to get back on your diet
- You can easily take on enough calories in one day to slow, stop or even reverse your weight loss

The optimum way to approach cheat days and meals is to experiment with them. See how your body reacts when you introduce one into your chosen nutritional plan and then adjust it based on how it works for you.

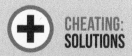

CHEATING:
SOLUTIONS

- *Cheat days are far harder to incorporate into a diet and still lose than cheat meals – you could even try two cheat meals per week, which has a better sense of balance than a day of total calorie annihilation (especially when you set the alarm clock for 00:01 to start gorging yourself).*
- *If you're cheating and not losing weight at the rate you want to, then you know where to start making the changes.*

MINDFUL EATING

Mindful eating is the process of being aware of what you are eating and taking the appropriate time to savour and enjoy your food. It's basically what your mum used to tell you to do – sit down when you're eating, chew your food slowly and don't just cram it in your mouth as fast as possible until you can see the pattern on the plate again. Obvious, right? Mindful eating is absolutely common sense but it's scary how far away we have strayed from the concept. Ever done any of these:

- Eating while watching TV or surfing the web? Not mindful eating.
- Eating while moving? Not mindful eating.
- Downing shots? Not mindful drinking.
- Only chewing enough so the food doesn't choke you? Not mindful eating.

A good way to approach mindful eating is to think of it as a perfect goal to aim for, but don't worry if you don't manage to achieve it at all times. This is the sort of thing that monks go and live in mountain-top temples to work on. You're leading a busy life, so it's enough to hold on to it as a concept and try to do these things at every meal:

- *Sit down to eat and focus on where you are and what's going on.*
- *Let eating and drinking be the only activity – switch off all other distractions.*
- *Take a deep breath before you start and be thankful.*
- *When you eat, chew slowly and notice the flavours, textures and smells of the food.*
- *Develop the skill of knowing when you feel full. It will always be sooner than you think.*

Mindful eating helps to connect you to your food in a way that will truly help you to appreciate and enjoy food more. It also helps your weight loss because by taking your time to eat your food you spend more time eating. It takes roughly 20 minutes for the stomach's 'full' signals to get to the brain and by that time, if you've been wolfing down the food, you could have taken in a huge amount of calories that you simply didn't need – or actually want.

HYDRATION

You are thirsty right now. According to one recent survey, over a third of men get less than the recommended levels of fluid in a day. Just as worrying is that for men aged between 19 and 64 only 21% of what they drank was water. If this is you, stop it. Or rather – start it. Not getting enough water is a fatal mistake when it comes to dieting. There are three reasons why:

- Eating because you're thirsty. The brain struggles to communicate the difference between thirst and hunger, all that it knows how to say is 'cram good stuff in your mouth'. It's not your fault if you're answering that call with biscuits, when actually what your body is saying is, 'I'm parched!'
- Dehydration manifests itself in funny ways. It's not just a dry mouth – studies have shown that you minus water equals more tension, anxiety and less concentration. All of those feelings can lead to emotional eating. Stop them before they happen by getting into good drinking habits.
- Your kidneys are responsible for filtering toxins out of your body, but when you are dehydrated this is much harder work.

Fortunately, keeping hydrated is just a habit, it's not difficult or complicated – just drink a lot more water on an ongoing basis. There's also a really simple and free way of checking your hydration levels: look at your urine. If you are adequately hydrated your urine should be the colour of light straw. If it's clear then you might be overly hydrated – anything that makes you think of dark yellows or highlighter pens should send you running towards the nearest tap – any other colours (browns, reds, blues) should send you to the doctor.

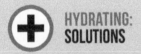

HYDRATING: SOLUTIONS

- *Drink a glass of water first thing in the morning before anything else. This gets you on your way to your hydration target but also moves your digestion along...*
- *Get a good water bottle you enjoy drinking out of and keep it with you whenever you're out. Just remember to clean it regularly.*
- *If you're one of the many men who simply find water boring check out our drinks recipes on page 236.*
- *Avoid the classic causes of dehydration: too much caffeine, alcohol, or very salty foods.*

INTERMITTENT FASTING

Intermittent Fasting (or IF) means reducing the period of time during a day when you consume your calories. Sometimes this means fasting for a whole day, but often this means only eating between the hours of 11am and 7pm if you are following a 16:8 pattern (16 hours fasting, 8 hours eating). Other patterns suggest anything up to 20 hours of fasting and then four hours where eating is allowed. The advantage of Intermittent Fasting is that it's really an add-on to any existing diet. But why would you bother – especially when you've always been told that skipping breakfast is a bad thing?

From a MAN v FAT point of view the prime reason is that after six to eight hours, your body's stores of energy from carbohydrates have been depleted and the body starts to metabolise fat. The other big benefit is that it's been shown that periods of fasting can boost levels of the Human Growth Hormone (responsible for building muscle and speeding up your metabolism) by up to 2,000% in men. There's also a psychological benefit from the controlled absence of food – although you don't feel hungry it does make you more aware, and thus more mindful, about what you are eating at other times.

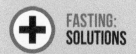

FASTING: SOLUTIONS

- *Make sure that Intermittent Fasting works for you by experimenting with it. Try a period of time that you feel will be comfortable and then plan your meals into a shorter timeframe.*
- *Ensure that your fast is at least 16 hours in length – this often means taking a late breakfast at 11am.*
- *Stick to your normal diet when you are eating – although some methods of Intermittent Fasting advocate eating whatever you want on the periods when you are not fasting, if you exceed your calorie limits then you will still gain weight.*

PROBIOTICS AND PREBIOTICS

The trend towards adding 'friendly bacteria' to our daily intake is a relatively recent phenomenon in the West, but it has been a mainstay of the cuisine and health regimes of other cultures for millennia. The confusion behind these probiotics and prebiotics arrives because we're often told that bacteria and germs are responsible for illnesses. This is certainly true, but it overlooks the fact that your body is a writhing battleground of bacteria. There are more bacteria in and on your body than human cells – in fact, 'You' are mostly bacteria. The theory is that, by adding 'good' bacteria to your gut (probiotics) and eating foods that support them (prebiotics), then you can create a more efficient digestive system, which amongst other benefits improves the uptake of nutrition from your food.

An example of this is the good bacteria lactobacillus, which changes the acid levels in your stomach and can prevent the growth of harmful bacteria. Studies have shown that adding bacteria like this into your gut can seriously reduce the impact of various illnesses, including Irritable Bowel Syndrome, as well as drastically reducing gut infections. There is a lot of research about how a more balanced digestive system can help to protect against Type 2 diabetes and obesity. Overall, this is definitely one to try out and monitor for a couple of months to see how it affects your own body.

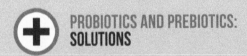

PROBIOTICS AND PREBIOTICS: SOLUTIONS

- *Good sources of probiotics and prebiotics include foods like sprouted vegetables, fermented vegetables, live yoghurts and drinks like kombucha and kefir (see page 236).*
- *Probiotics and prebiotics are particularly important if you are taking a course of antibiotics as these can seriously reduce the number of good bacteria in your gut, meaning that you will need to replace them as soon as possible.*

MEDITATION AND BREATHING TECHNIQUES

Regardless of whether the stress or anxiety in your life is putting you under too much pressure, there are a number of ways that incorporating meditation into your routine and practising breathing techniques can help with your weight loss. Primarily these include lowering your blood pressure and cortisol levels, clearing the mind and helping you to quieten and control your thoughts. Losing weight and following a diet can put extra pressure on your life and consequently taking steps to help stay calm and focused is always a good investment of your time.

SQUARE BREATHING

The simplest form of breathing training can be done in just about any situation or setting. It's also a technique that is taught to soldiers to help them keep focused and relaxed in difficult situations – if it works for someone who is being shot at then there's a good chance it will work for you too.

Find somewhere comfortable to sit or kneel and close your eyes. Imagine a square in front of you. Each side of the square will represent an inhalation, a pause, an exhalation or a pause. Start with a count of four. When you breathe in, try and imagine you are inflating a balloon in your stomach; as you breathe out, allow the air to flow out of your stomach.

- Breathe in for a steady count of four.
- Hold the breath in for a steady count of four.
- Slowly release the breath for a steady count of four.
- Hold the breath out for a count of four.

Don't worry if you find holding the breath in and holding it out feels unnatural – it will at first. If the count is too long, then simply reduce it to two. Complete 10 trips around the square. As you progress, simply lengthen the time for each section of the square. By the time you get to a steady count of eight you should find that your ability to control your breath is improving drastically.

ALTERNATE NOSTRIL BREATHING

Also known to yogis as Nadi Shodhana, this may seem a bit strange at first, especially if you've got a cold, but stick with it and you'll find that it's incredibly effective at calming the mind and body and releasing tension.

Find somewhere comfortable to sit or kneel. Using the thumb of your right hand, push on the outside of your right nostril so only your left nostril is open. Inhale through your left nostril for a count of four. At the top of the breath, switch sides. Use the little finger of the right hand to close off the left nostril and steadily exhale through the right nostril for a steady count of four. Then inhale through the right nostril for a count of four, close off the right nostril with the thumb and exhale through the left nostril for a steady count of four.

Repeat this process for up to five cycles of breathing. If you feel comfortable, attempt to increase the length of the steady count that you inhale and exhale for.

PROGRESSIVE RELAXATION

This is another simple-to-master but incredibly effective technique that is perfect for relaxation, stress relief or preparation for a good night's sleep. It requires you to find somewhere comfortable to sit, or preferably lie down. Focusing on different body parts at each breath, you are going to breathe in and hold the breath for a steady count of five, before exhaling. Do this three times to get comfortable with the pattern.

On the fourth inhale, contract the muscles of your feet (tense your toes, your ankles and soles of your feet as hard as you can) for the full count of five. When you breathe out, release the muscles completely and allow them to let go. On the next hold, tense the muscles around your shins and calves. Again when you breathe out relax them completely. Work your way through the body following the same pattern:

- Feet
- Shins and calves
- Thighs and buttocks
- Stomach and lower back
- Chest and lungs
- Hands and wrists
- Arms
- Shoulders
- Neck and chin
- Face
- Skull

Once you get to the top of your head you should return to three full breaths with no contraction or squeezing. Enjoy the feeling of complete relaxation and heaviness that now exists in your body.

MEDITATION

There are many different kinds of meditation from Transcendental to Christian but all of them revolve around the principle of stilling the mind through calm posture and a focus on the breathing. For a simple beginner's session, try a three-minute period of sitting calmly with your eyes shut, no distractions and focusing solely on your breath. Thoughts will come into your head but don't hold on to them. Simply allow them to drift from your mind and focus on your breathing.

In partnership with square breathing practice this can be incredibly powerful, even for a three-minute spell. As you get into the practice try and extend the time that you meditate for sessions of up to 10 minutes or longer. Some people find that it helps to focus on a mantra or a message – a simple truth or positive thought (possibly related to your weight loss) that you allow yourself to repeat in your mind. If you find your mind has wandered, don't get annoyed or feel like you're failing, simply return to your chosen thought or clear your mind entirely and focus on your breathing. If you would like to experiment more with meditation look at **www.manvfat.com/resources**.

SUPPLEMENTS AND VITAMINS

The key issue here is that you understand that there are no magic pills when it comes to weight loss – despite what the manufacturers' marketing materials say and however plausible the bloke at the gym sounds. For the same reason that this book doesn't discuss gastric bands as a weight-loss option, neither are we looking at the medically prescribed weight-loss drugs. This is because ultimately the responsibility to lose weight is about you changing your own eating and activity habits. Outsourcing the responsibility to a pill or an operation will not teach you how to eat and be active for the rest of your life and could lead to disappointment and unnecessary health risks.

That said, there are a range of supplements that you should consider adding to your daily intake. Nutritional deficiencies are as real as the symptoms they produce and although most of the issues will be solved by a healthy, balanced diet, supplements can be a useful addition. As long as they're not going to clash with any medications you are on and you are happy to accept the cost then there is little danger in experimenting with a wide range of supplements and vitamins and seeing which ones make you feel better.

For example, I know that there's not much evidence to suggest that wheatgrass is an effective addition to a healthy lifestyle but I still drink it – in part because it tastes so comically bad (imagine a plant farting in your mouth) that everything else tastes great by comparison, but also because it makes me 'feel' more energised. It's almost certainly a placebo effect, but there are days when I really don't care! Here are five common deficiencies that you might want to address through dietary changes or supplements. Always consult your doctor if you have symptoms you're concerned about and ask them to OK any new vitamins or supplements you're adding to your routine – just brace yourself for some scepticism!

1. IRON

Over 30% of the world's population are anaemic (iron deficient). Get a blood test to determine if you are.

SYMPTOMS: Fatigue, palpitations, pale complexion, desire to eat non-food items (such as ice). Vegans and vegetarians are more prone to anaemia, but carnivores are still at risk.

TREATMENT: Dietary changes, including avoiding tea and eating more dark green leafy vegetables with butter (like kale and watercress). Improve your Vitamin C levels to help absorb iron. Iron supplements such as Floradix or Spatone can be helpful.

2. VITAMIN D

A lack of exposure to natural sunlight and poor diet have led to over 1 billion people worldwide being deficient.

SYMPTOMS: Primarily fatigue, but Vitamin D helps your body to absorb calcium, so a deficiency will mean weaker bones and teeth.

TREATMENT: Speak to a doctor to get your levels tested. They will prescribe supplements and advise on lifestyle changes that can help to address it. In addition get out into the fresh air as often as possible.

3. MAGNESIUM

One report stated that up to 20% of all hospital patients and up to 65% of intensive care patients are magnesium deficient.

SYMPTOMS: Possible link to migraines, diabetes and hypertension. A very common symptom is muscle twitches around the eyes and in the legs. There are also links to atrial fibrillation.

TREATMENT: You will need to ask a doctor to specifically test for magnesium levels but if you suspect you are deficient, try adding cashews and almonds, fresh coconut, spinach and high-quality dark chocolate to your diet. Alternatively, add magnesium to your daily supplements.

4. VITAMIN B12

This deficiency becomes more common as you age, with over 20% showing a marginal deficiency after 60 years of age.

SYMPTOMS: Perhaps the most alarming side effect here is the possible link to dementia and reduced cognitive function. Early signals can be tingling in the fingers or a ringing in the ears.

TREATMENT: Adding shellfish, liver, milk and yogurt to your diet can all help; alternatively talk to your doctor about supplementing.

5. OMEGA 3

An essential fatty acid and a boost in fighting cardiovascular disease.

SYMPTOMS: We all need Omega 3 in our diet and if you don't eat much fatty fish (that's salmon, mackerel or sardines) then you could find yourself coming up short. Omega 3s have been shown to be effective in helping with cardiovascular disease and even low moods.

TREATMENT: You should try and get at least two 75g servings of fatty fish per week, or supplement with high-quality Omega 3 tablets every day.

CHRIS EICHFELD

Age: 39 **Job:** Corporate purchasing for Five Guys Burgers and Fries
Height: 6' (182cm) **Heaviest weight:** 321.9lb (146kg)
Lowest weight: 170lb (77.1kg)

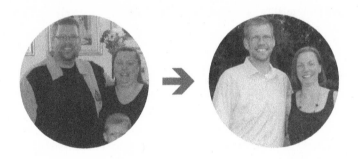

I'd always been a chubby kid. I had asthma and my father smoked so we had a lot of second-hand smoke in the house and I always had bronchitis. Consequently, running and exercise weren't easy. I was never overly good at sports, so there was just food. The way we ate as a family was always a meat, a potato and then a starchy vegetable covered in butter. My father, my mother, my sister were all overweight. We were just a fat family. We were your typical American fat family.

For years my wife and I wanted to get healthy – we just never had the motivation. We had a gym membership and never went. My wife got pregnant so we said, 'Oh, we have to stay and look after the baby.' Then we got an elliptical trainer for the house – which became a clothes rack! Plus, I work in the food industry and I love cooking. I always said it would be great to get healthy and then never did anything about it. I think for men we struggle because of our egos. I think we have a hard time communicating feelings and personal struggles. It's a lot easier to joke and laugh and say, 'Ha ha, I'm the fat guy!' as opposed to saying, 'Hey, I don't want to be this person any more.'

My wife and I both did Weight Watchers and in terms of the practicalities I did the whole thing online. My wife did online with the meetings. I just couldn't bring myself to go and sit and talk about being overweight. My wife was very successful with the meetings. She enjoys that support structure and she enjoys listening to everyone else and their challenges. That helped motivate her, but for me it was watching the weight come off.

In my opinion, Weight Watchers' points structure is probably the best thing going, knowing you've got your limits, but when you start it's very high. It's not daunting, they're not setting you up for failure. When the weight started coming off easily I thought, I can do this. What helped for me was that fruits and unprocessed vegetables are zero points, so you can snack on those all the time. I can eat those all day, every day. If I'm hungry and I need to snack, I go get a piece of fruit or get some veg. The weight loss actually came easily, it wasn't as big of a challenge as I thought it would be.

I more or less halved my body weight, so when I lost the weight people I hadn't seen for a while just had no idea it was me. That was the strangest thing. Then of course people want to congratulate you but then they think you're sick. I had someone come up to me and go, 'You're not dying, are you?' I said, 'No!' They said, 'In which case, great job on losing weight!'

My advice would be that you have to want it, and you have to want it for yourself. So many people say they're doing it for someone else and you just can't. You have to do it for you. I look back and I realise I was angry about my weight. There is a sense of being comfortable in your own skin when you lose weight. If you're not comfortable in your own skin then you'll make everyone else around you miserable.

I would also say you have to set manageable goals. I started out and I said OK – let me get below 300lb (136kg). That was 20lb (9kg). Then I said – let me hit 270. 250. Let me make it 210 and I will have lost 100lb (45kg)! Then I thought it would be great to be under 200lb (91kg). If you find something that works for you – stick with it! Don't get frustrated – if it's not working, go back and see what was working and do more of that. Finally, I'd say you have to find a support system. I didn't do the meetings but I had my wife. We ate the same foods and we could talk to each other and share ideas, so don't be afraid to ask for help.

www.manvfat.com/members/cwbooyakasha

MARK SOSENE

Age: 36 **Job:** Data specialist **Height:** 5'11" (181cm)
Heaviest weight: 339.5lb (154kg) **Lowest weight:** 207.2lb (94kg)

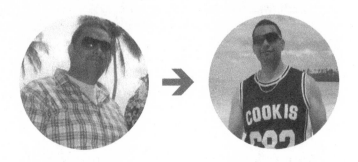

A few years ago I noticed I was always tired, really completely lethargic, and I was thirsty a lot. Of course back then when I was thirsty I would grab a Coke, I hardly drank water. At times I was starting to get dizzy as well. I saw the doctor and he said that all of these things I was experiencing were down to my weight. My blood pressure was sky high, I was borderline diabetic and I couldn't sleep. I was a mess.

My grandparents brought me up, they were like my mum and dad, and so when my Granddad had his heart attack and died that was a big thing for me. I'm the oldest in my generation and I looked at my little brothers and sisters and my cousins and suddenly the responsibility just struck me – what kind of a message am I sending them if I don't get myself sorted? And don't I want to get fit and healthy and live a full life?

The Cook Islands, where I'm from, has one of the worst obesity rates in the world. 92% of people there are obese and it's shocking. Quite simply it's easier and cheaper to buy junk food. There's also a culture of eating big portions there; like on Sunday we'll go to church and come home and the table will be absolutely full of food. Then you've got your grandmother going, 'You can't leave the table until you've finished – and don't you want dessert?'

I was fat because I was drinking too much. I would work throughout the week and Friday night I would always go out and wouldn't go home! I'd recover all day Saturday and then go out again. Don't get me wrong – I had an awesome time, but it affects your health. And of course the bad foods go hand in hand with the bad drinking. When you're hungry at midnight there are no salad stores open.

Previously, I'd done Weight Watchers and Jenny Craig and those hadn't worked for me. This time I decided I'd figure out my own system. I knew that the two things I had to do were to get my eating under control and get into exercise. I solved the food issue by getting MyFitnessPal and using calories as a guide to work out how much I should be eating and what foods. I decided that I'd stop drinking alcohol and allow myself one cheat day a week for take-out.

It was hard at the start trying to work out what food worked for me and experimenting with how much exercise to do. But I read a lot, asked questions and worked out the answers. After that it was a case of having a positive mindset and being patient. I set small weekly and monthly targets and the positivity really paid off when I had a plateau after two months. I figured out that I needed to change my exercise routine and I had to be really patient with myself because I wanted fast results.

When I was big I didn't like gyms, I didn't feel comfortable there and I realised I would rather exercise in my own home, so I bought a treadmill. I made sure I put it right in front of the TV, so I had to do it every day. I also decorated it with a photo of my granddad and a lot of inspiring pictures, quotes and messages so if I looked at that I couldn't be sitting on the couch. When I first started I could hardly do anything on it. But I stuck with it. Every day I got back on it and tried a little harder and went a little further. Over time my legs gained muscle and the weight started to drop off.

When I saw the doctor after I lost weight he said, 'How the hell have you done that?' He was thrilled. He said that the weight had come off at the right rate – it took about two years in total. Though I really hate needles, I didn't mind having a blood test after I'd reached my goal weight and all the results for thyroid function, diabetes and blood pressure were normal. It was so cool seeing that by taking control of what I was eating I'd managed to save my body from all of those illnesses, and you can do it too.
www.manvfat.com/members/mark-sosene

STEP THREE:
CREATE A WINNING STRUCTURE

SKIP THIS STEP IF:

- You want your weight loss to fail

"Perfect planning prevents piss-poor performance."

Army saying

SPOILER WARNING:

Like all of the spoilers so far in this book, this one comes right from the Central Bureau of the Blindingly Obvious, but it's so often overlooked by men when it comes to diets that it's worth re-stating: Unless you plan and structure your weight-loss efforts correctly then you will NOT succeed.

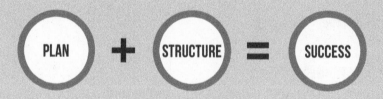

One of the key reasons for diets failing is that they start on a surge of determination. Perhaps you've just seen a photo of you that has given you a much-needed slap in the face and you're determined to make a change. We want that change to happen now, so we make a quick decision about what diet to do, research the absolute basics about how it works and trust that our determination will see us through.

But as the shock of the photo recedes and is replaced by the shock of your new extreme eating and exercise plan, very soon your resolve wavers. Perhaps you get drunk, or break your diet rules. Possibly both. Then the spiral of anger and emotional eating starts and, before you know it, you've put the weight back on. Sound familiar to you?

Not this time.

This time – no matter what diet or activity you've chosen from Step Two and whatever reason you've been working on for being fat from Step One – this time you're going to do it right and that means creating a winning structure. The following Step contains lots of actions and preparations. If it takes a week to undertake this preparation then by all means carry on eating and drinking in your normal way while you get ready. It's more important that when you make a change you do so with all the groundwork in place – forget to dig out the foundations and see how long a building lasts...

Creating a winning structure consists of five steps:

(1) SETTING YOUR GOALS

(2) GETTING EQUIPPED

(3) IDENTIFYING THREATS AND SUPPORT

(4) TRACKING AND REVIEWING YOUR PROGRESS

(5) CHANGING YOUR MINDSET

SETTING YOUR GOALS

This is the fun part of planning; it's where you make decisions about who you want to become on the other side of your weight loss. There are so many different methods of setting your goals and ultimately it's a very personal thing – you might be more driven by your appearance, or perhaps you simply want to get better at sport. An essential question to ask yourself when setting your goals is whether you really want these things for you. When you look at your goals and motivations, are they things that other people want from you, or are they things that come from your heart? The strongest goals – the ones that will keep you motivated during the hard times – are the ones that you want to achieve for yourself.

Having a range of goals from a number of different angles stops you focusing on one particular aspect of weight loss. For example, it may well be that one week the scales report no change to your weight but you're able to fit into a shirt that was previously too tight for you, or you can now complete Phase Two of the walking fitness plan. You could get demoralised if weight loss was your only goal, but seeing the wider picture with a range of goals can help you to stay positive.

So let's set some goals.

 TIP *The more detailed and specific you can make your goals the stronger they will be and the easier it will be to track your progress.*

GOAL #1
WHAT DO YOU WANT TO WEIGH?

Body Mass Index (BMI) is one of the main weight metrics used by medical professionals around the world and is calculated on your weight and height. Your BMI reading is split into a range of categories:

- BMI under 18.5 – Underweight
- BMI 18.5 to 25 – Healthy range
- BMI 25 to 30 – Overweight
- BMI 30 or over – Obese

There are plenty of arguments against BMI as a good measure (it doesn't work so well if you're very tall, or carry a lot of muscle) so take it with a pinch of a low-sodium salt alternative. However, it can be a reasonable starting point for setting a target weight, or as the 'joke' goes – a target height. You can get this quickly and easily by filling out your Health Report at **www.manvfat.com/healthreport**.

MY GOAL WEIGHT IS:

GOAL #2
WHAT DO YOU WANT TO LOOK LIKE?

We might not openly admit it but how we look is a big concern for men and it can have a huge impact on how you feel, which is often linked to your confidence in any situation – and your happiness. I've split this appearance goal into three different metrics – your personal goal, your body measurements and your body fat percentage.

1. PERSONAL GOAL

When you set your personal goal you should be as specific as possible. It also helps if you can phrase this particular target in terms of negatives and positives. So not only should you state what you want to move away from, you should also state what you want to move towards. For example, if there are parts of your body that you dislike then you should specify these negatives, but you should also register some positives you're aiming for, too – perhaps you have a very specific shirt you want to fit into and feel confident wearing.

MY APPEARANCE GOAL NEGATIVE IS:
What do you want to move away from?

_____

_____

MY APPEARANCE GOAL POSITIVE IS:
What do you want to move towards?

_____

_____

2. BODY MEASUREMENTS

When you lose weight and start to become more active your body shape will change. There are a number of ways available to you to monitor your body shape – including expensive options such as DEXA scans (a type of X-ray that gives a picture of the body's make up). It's important to have the ability to check your progress regularly, though – so although you might want to book in for a scan at different stages of your weight loss, simple body measurements are a reliable and free way of understanding how your body shape is changing. For this you will need a tape measure – see page 171.

Measuring your body often requires more than two hands. Recruit a volunteer – just make sure you know them!

Let it all hang out. There's no point measuring your belly while you're sucking it in – get the worst-case scenario and see your body for how it really is.

WHERE AND HOW TO MEASURE:

- **Chest**

Finally a reason for men to have nipples – they're the perfect visual marker for where you should measure your chest. Wrap the tape measure around your chest, keep your arms relaxed by your side and record.

_____

- **Belly button**

Again another very simple way of keeping your measurement in the same place every time you measure. Record your waist size.

_____

- **Bicep**

Around the widest part of your arm when your bicep is flexed – do both left and right and record.

_____

- **Thigh**

Choose the widest part of your thigh, measure both legs and record.

_____

These measurements can give you a total picture and, measured on a fortnightly or monthly basis, you should be able to see some real inches lost. With body measurements you won't have a fixed goal of where you want to end up, but just knowing that you've lost inches can be very motivating.

3. BODY-FAT PERCENTAGE

As the name would suggest this is a measure of what percentage of your body is made up of fat. This is an important thing to know because it's possible to be obese according to your BMI and yet have a very low body-fat percentage. Unfortunately, we can put a man on the moon but technology has yet to give us a way of reliably measuring body fat at home. Therefore the rule with body fat is to take a measurement each month and accept that it will fluctuate by as much as 5–10%.

A good hand-held model like the Omron body composition monitors will give you a good idea of what percentage of your body is fat. You can also get a pair of callipers and measure your own body fat by hand (the technique for doing this will vary depending on the model). Again the point to bear in mind is that your body fat is only really useful as a long-term metric. A very general guide for body fat is to say that:

30%+ large gut, man-boobs
20–30% small gut, few bits that jiggle
10–20% no gut, better definition of muscles
Under 10% no gut, no jiggling, 'ripped'

The chart below outlines exactly what your body fat target should be:

AGE	BODY FAT % MEASUREMENT CHART							
18 -20	2.0	3.9	6.2	8.5	10.5	12.5	14.3	16.0
21-25	2.5	4.9	7.3	9.5	11.6	13.6	15.4	17.0
26-30	3.5	6.0	8.4	10.6	12.7	14.6	16.4	18.1
31-35	4.5	7.1	9.4	11.7	13.7	15.7	17.5	19.2
36-40	5.6	8.1	10.5	12.7	14.8	16.8	18.6	20.2
41-45	6.7	9.2	11.5	13.8	15.9	17.8	19.6	21.3
46-50	7.7	10.2	12.6	14.8	16.9	18.9	20.7	22.4
51-55	8.8	11.3	13.7	15.9	18.0	20.0	21.8	23.4
56 & Up	9.9	12.4	14.7	17.0	19.1	21.0	22.8	24.5

LEAN   IDEAL

GOAL #3
WHAT DO YOU WANT TO BE ABLE TO DO?

Ask yourself this question and think seriously about the answer – what do you really want to do in your life and does your current body shape and level of fitness allow you to do that to the best of your ability? It can be so easy to become divorced from our real goals when we put on weight that this question might be tough for you to answer – it could be that you've hidden your fitness ambitions away because you would feel ridiculous even saying them to yourself. This is where you dust them off and declare them.

Understand that your body is a tool which is capable of incredible things – currently you might find that difficult to see, but simply by stating your fitness and health goals you start the journey to achieving them. It might seem like your heart's desire to run a marathon is so absurd you couldn't possibly even say it aloud – but here and now declare what it is that you want to achieve without any fear or embarrassment. Other aims might be more simple: to be able to play with your kids in the park, to set a good example to friends or family, to achieve a particular dream such as climbing a mountain, or swimming with whales,

BODY FAT % MEASUREMENT CHART

17.5	18.9	20.2	21.3	22.3	23.1	23.8	24.3	24.9
18.6	20.0	21.2	22.3	23.3	24.2	24.9	25.4	25.8
19.6	21.0	22.3	23.4	24.4	25.2	25.9	26.5	26.9
20.7	22.1	23.4	24.5	25.5	26.3	27.0	27.5	28.0
21.8	23.2	24.4	25.6	26.5	27.4	28.1	28.6	29.0
22.8	24.7	25.5	26.6	27.6	28.4	29.1	29.7	30.1
23.9	25.3	26.6	27.7	28.7	29.5	30.2	30.7	31.2
25.0	26.4	27.6	28.7	29.7	30.6	31.2	31.8	32.2
26.0	27.4	28.7	29.8	30.8	31.6	32.3	32.9	33.3

AVERAGE   **ABOVE AVERAGE**

to beat diabetes... It doesn't matter how bonkers you think it is right now – write out your health goals here.

MY HEALTH AND FITNESS GOALS ARE:

_____

_____

_____

_____

_____

_____

_____

_____

CHECKLIST:
YOUR COMPLETE GOAL LIST SHOULD NOW HAVE

☐ **WEIGHT**

☐ **APPEARANCE**

☐ **HEALTH AND FITNESS**

BREAKING YOUR GOALS DOWN

Your goals are the ultimate tool in motivating your weight loss. However, unless you use them in the right way they could actually be damaging. When you're driving a long distance you'll know just how depressing it can be to follow your progress on a map. It feels like you're crawling along at a snail's pace – and then when you look at how far you've got to go, it can be enough to make you want to turn around and go back. It's the same with your weight-loss goals.

The key is to split all of your goals down into smaller steps. Between the three categories of goals you'll then have a number of smaller targets that you can group into as many mini-goals as you require. Let's take the example of weight – if you weigh 315lb (143kg) and you want to reach 215lb (97kg) then you could split the overall goal up into ten mini-goals of 10lb (4.5kg). Alternatively, you might decide to look at a 'major milestones' approach and have four mini-goals at 300lb, 275, 250 and 225. So long as each mini-goal is within sight and you keep things realistic and achievable then you can break it down however you like.

REWARDS

Hitting your goals and mini-goals, losing weight and feeling healthier is its own reward, but it never hurts to give yourself an added incentive of a reward at various points along your weight-loss journey.

 The best rewards are not food- or drink-related! In fact, for an extra kick, make your rewards boost your journey towards a healthier you. How about the following ideas:

- New trainers or sports gear
- Entry into a race or fitness event
- Buy new clothes and declutter your wardrobe of items that are starting to feel too big

- Get a personal shopper to advise you on wearing the right clothes for your new body shape
- Attend to an element of your appearance you'd like to improve – e.g. teeth whitening or getting a tattoo (or having one removed!)
- Gym membership or personal training sessions
- A wearable fitness tracker, heart rate monitor or other sports equipment
- Cinema trips
- New music or books
- For every pound lost add money to a jar which is 'unlocked' as you hit your goals
- A photo-shoot showing off your new look – use it to update your social media profiles and your ID cards – start to erase the old fat you
- A massage, reflexology or treatment of your choice
- New vitamins or supplements
- Travel somewhere you always wanted to go
- Donation to charity

Break your three goals down into mini-goals here using the table on the right (you can also find printable charts at **www.manvfat.com/resources**).

TIMING YOUR GOALS

You will now have a list of lots of goals for your weight-loss journey, which have been broken down into a number of mini-goals, and you have a clear idea of what the rewards are along the way. Now, comes the vexed issue of timing – how long is it going to take for you to hit these goals?

The absolute best advice is **FORGET ABOUT HOW LONG IT WILL TAKE.** Think about all of the disappointments surrounding diets – if it's not because your new diet isn't working, it's nearly always because things haven't gone according to the timescale you've imagined.

MY GOALS AND REWARDS	WEIGHT GOAL	APPEARANCE GOAL	HEALTH & FITNESS GOAL
Mini Goal 1			
Reward			
Mini Goal 2			
Reward			
Mini Goal 3			
Reward			
Ultimate Goal			
Ultimate Reward			

The truth is that weight loss isn't a precise science. Sometimes things go slowly, sometimes they go faster. It's guaranteed that at some point during your weight loss things will go absolutely nowhere – maybe even for a few weeks. By all means try to reach your goals as quickly as is safely possible – but don't say that your diet will have been a failure unless you reach a certain goal within X months. Remember that the 'six-pack in six weeks' has always been a con – DON'T fall for it.

 For a healthy and happy weight loss, know what your goals are, know what the rewards are and let the timing go.

For clarity, this isn't the same thing as saying that you shouldn't measure your progress; you absolutely *must* track how your diet is going. If you insist on putting a timescale to your weight loss then you should consider that, on average, 1–2lb (0.5–1kg) a week is a very reasonable amount to lose. In the earlier stages of weight loss, or if you have a lot to lose, then you might experience anywhere up to 10lb (4.5kg) loss per week, but this is way above average and will not remain at this rate – expecting any more will result in disappointment. When planning the timing of weight loss always allow for one week out of four to maintain weight, which accounts for things like holidays and periods of illness.

GETTING EQUIPPED

By 2017, the weight-loss market is expected to be worth $361 billion. That's a lot of Thighmasters. But for every gadget that helps you to lose weight, there are countless others that will simply be relegated to the loft of shame and provide an amusing home for spiders. Getting the structure of your diet right means that you will have to equip yourself with everything you need to make it work.

FOOD AND DRINK

This may seem like an obvious one but you are going to need to buy in food and drink for you to consume during your diet. The best way to prepare for this is to research the sort of foods and meals you will be eating on your diet (see diet reviews on pages 69–99). In researching your particular diet you should be able to put together at least a fortnight's menu plan (but preferably a month's) which fits in with your diet.

You should plan at least five:

- Breakfasts
- Lunches
- Dinners
- Snacks
- Drinks
- Emergency meals (i.e. what you will eat if you can't follow your plan for any reason)
- Treats/Cheats

Although this might seem like a lot of work, it is essential preparation. Not only will it enable you to check that your intake matches the particular diet you are doing, it will also give you a head-start when it comes to shopping for food. You can plan so that there is far less wastage across the week (so that leftover roast dinners from Sunday become leftover casseroles early in the week) and you will also be able to shop to a very strict list. That reduces the impulse purchases that deviate from the principles of what you're doing.

TIP *Doing your food shopping online might cost you more in delivery but you save on travel to the supermarket and time, while often discount vouchers allow you to recoup the delivery fee. You also avoid impulse purchases or overfilling your trolley because you're tired, you're hungry or tempted by marketing.*

Planning ahead in terms of food is also useful because it helps to give you a picture of what you will be eating on the diet and allows you to master the little tricks and cheats which will keep things interesting (searching on **www.manvfat.com/ diets** is a good shortcut to finding ideas for different meals on any given diet). Contemplating your plan can be a shortcut to realising that there are significant problems with your intended diet. Realising that you'll need to eat chilli every meal when you hate kidney beans could be all of the incentive you need to find a more varied programme.

Herbs, spices and condiments like chilli sauce, soy sauce and ginger are allowed on most diets – learn to use them properly and love them because between them they can make any meal edible. Go for fresh herbs where possible and know that grinding your own spices with a pestle and mortar hugely improves the flavour. Beware of other condiments like tomato ketchup or barbecue sauce, which can be very heavily processed and full of sugars. In combination with other 'unseen dangers' these can really undermine your weight loss.

TIP *Don't assume – make sure that the meals you plan really do fit in with your chosen diet, including if you need to weigh ingredients. Making even a small mistake when you set off could lead to you going miles off track as your diet progresses.*

Depending on who you live with this next step might not be possible but it's advisable to purge your house of foods that don't fit with what you're doing. Depending on your willpower you might like to make sure that you don't have quantities of biscuits, cakes and crisps to hand – which you could turn to in a moment of weakness. If this causes friction then you have already identified one possible threat to your diet (see page 176).

WEIGHT-LOSS EQUIPMENT

There are very few pieces of equipment that could be considered essential to weight loss. Depending on your budget many of these can be borrowed or accessed in other places (doctor's surgeries or gyms for scales and body fat monitors, for example). In which case you shouldn't consider this an essential shopping list – more a list of items that all have value when it comes to losing weight, regardless of which diet you end up choosing.

1 SMARTPHONES

If you were looking for a reason to upgrade your old Nokia 5110 then weight loss is a great one. Smartphones have GPS, the magic of the internet and a wealth of weight-loss apps which means that your phone can track you on bike rides, tell you how many calories are in a pint of Stella (256) and even give you access to the monthly MAN v FAT magazine.

2 TAPE MEASURES

Although specialised weight-loss tape measures do exist, they're mostly gimmicky nonsense. Stick with a simple tailor's tape measure (not a retractable builder's tape measure!). They're cheap, don't stretch and will do the job perfectly – just remember where to take the measurements (see page 160).

3 BODY FAT MEASURES

You can either use hand-held callipers which are used to pinch the skin at various points around the body and give you a reading of body-fat percentage, or you can use an electronic body-fat measurer which sends a pulse of electricity painlessly through the body to calculate your body fat. The hand-held versions are simpler and give a good overall sense of your body-fat levels provided you follow the instructions and don't assume that they give you an exact measurement.

4 SCALES

You want digital scales that are accurate and that go up to your weight, as many stop at 400lb (183kg). The modern brand of wifi scales will connect to your home network and update apps that you link to your account. It's a gimmicky feature but it's fun to have and if you are invested in a particular system to track your measurements it can save time. Ultimately, though, spend money on a more accurate pair of scales as this is the most important element.

5 WATER BOTTLES

Choose a water bottle you love and you're more likely to drink from it and remember to bring it with you. Camelbak make great, no-spill models and if you're the forgetful type then try a Hydracoach. New smart cups like Vessyl, which automatically calculate the calories and nutritional elements of any drink you put in them, are an interesting development but perhaps at too early a stage to qualify as an essential purchase.

TIP *See drinks recipes on page 236 for some ideas on healthy drinks and making hydration less of a chore.*

6 HAND BLENDERS

Soups are brilliant for weight loss; they're filling, you can cram as much veg into them as you like and when they're liquidised they all taste more palatable. A good hand blender should also be able to create a morning smoothie as well.

7 MEASURING SPOONS

Accuracy of measurements is essential – although it won't completely derail your diet, knowing the difference between a tablespoonful and a teaspoonful can save a huge amount of calories across a year.

8 ZIPLOCK BAGS AND TUPPERWARE

Get good strong ziplock bags and a range of Tupperware containers. That means you will always have access to your own snacks if you're at the cinema, and you'll have a storage solution for all your cooking, leftovers and packed-lunch needs. Boring, maybe. Essential, definitely.

9 SMALLER PLATES

This is always one of the laughable cheats given to dieters – eat off a small plate and you'll think you're having a bigger portion! As if! It really does work though and giving yourself any advantage you can on your diet is a good idea.

10 GRATERS

You might well have an ordinary grater at home but get a Microplane grater and you'll love it for ever. Why does it help? Research has found that people believe they're served nearly 50% more of a food when it's shredded. Equally, you'll save calories – for example a cup of grated cheese contains around 70 calories fewer than a cup of the cubed variety.

11 PESTLES AND MORTARS

Get a pestle and mortar and you'll be able to spice up your foods in no time. If you've never eaten roasted mushrooms with freshly ground cumin then you've never lived.

12 JUICERS

It's impossible to escape the fact that juicing is in vogue at the moment, but you should see it as a part of a healthy lifestyle and a good way to get a range of vitamins and minerals into your daily routine, not as the exclusive answer to your weight loss. The Philips range are reasonably priced and perform well.

13 WEARABLE FITNESS TRACKERS

In a few years, wearable trackers will be everything we hope they are today, but the current generation of models are limited if you're looking for something that monitors sleep, exercise and heart rate. So for now the best thing to do is go for something simple that works reliably. The Vivofit from Garmin is brilliant – it's a watch that nags you to move and counts how many steps you take. Plus it's waterproof, syncs easily and the battery lasts an entire year.

14 HEART RATE MONITORS

There are various 'sweet spots' on the heart rate scale which show you when you are in the perfect zone for burning fat. The reason heart rate monitors aren't that essential is because you are a very good judge of how hard your heart is working. The Rate of Perceived Exertion scale – where you take a guess on a scale of 1–10 how hard you're working – has been shown to be accurate, and it can be tested using the Talk Test (see page 113).

15 TRAINERS

You'll notice that there's very little exercise equipment on this list. This is because you really don't actually need much equipment at all to exercise. Somewhere to move and your own body weight is more than enough. However, what goes on your feet is vital. You should look for a shop that offers gait analysis so they can see what your feet are up to as you move and recommend a pair of trainers that are going to support you. Better trainer, fewer injuries, more enjoyable exercise – it's that simple.

WHAT YOUR FEET MEAN FOR YOU AND EXERCISE

FLAT FEET

If your feet have no arches, or 'fallen arches' as the condition is more commonly described, then you can be said to have 'flat feet'. If you are flat-footed, you're likely to overpronate, which means that your feet roll inward and your weight is not distributed evenly when you walk or run. This can put a strain on your muscles and ligaments, which may cause pain in your legs when you walk. If you're an overpronator getting into running, you may wish to invest in stabilising running shoes and even shoe inserts that can correct your gait, known as orthotics. Stretching your calf and Achilles tendon may also help as a tight Achilles can make your foot overpronate.

HIGH ARCHES

A high instep is less common than flat feet, but can be recognised as a very distinct hollow region between the ball and heel when the foot is bearing weight. If you have high arches, you are more likely to supinate or underpronate, which means your feet roll outwards as you walk or run. Again, the strengthening of a tight or weak Achilles tendon, along with the use of orthotics and specialised cushioned footwear, can help distribute weight more evenly and relieve the stress.

NEUTRAL ARCHES

If your arches are neither high nor fallen, you have normal, or 'neutral' feet. Your gait should naturally curve inward, but you shouldn't find that you overpronate. Providing you don't wear shoes that alter your gait, you should find your weight is distributed evenly when walking or running and the only pain you experience will be as a result of overall excess weight.

IDENTIFYING THREATS AND SUPPORT

Consider this quotation from Jim Rohn: 'You are the average of the five people you spend the most time with.' Write out who those five people are for you – we've filled in the first one for you:

1 – Yourself
_____

2
_____

3
_____

4
_____

5
_____

When you look at who those people are and you consider what the average of those five people would look like – does it start to give you a clearer picture of why you are where you are? Before you start to panic and think that we're going to tell you to leave your partner, get rid of your friends and divorce your family, understand that the problem may not lie with those people, but could instead lie with how you communicate your desire to be healthier to them. After all, if they don't know that you want support achieving something, how can they be blamed for not giving you that help? In the Big Fat Survey we asked people to specify if there was anyone who didn't support their weight loss. The results are surprising.

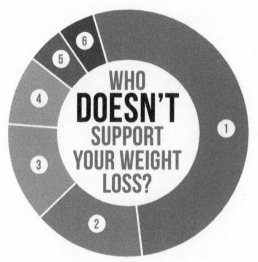

1. **EVERYONE SUPPORTS ME** 53%
2. **ME** 15%
3. **PARTNER** 13%
4. **WORK COLLEAGUES** 9%
5. **FRIENDS** 5%
6. **FAMILY** 5%

The great thing about this is that the majority of men feel that everyone gives them the support that they're looking for. If you feel the same that doesn't mean you can skip this section – there are ways of turning those supporters into ultra-supporters.

Perhaps the biggest surprise is seeing how many men were aware that they were the one who didn't support their weight loss. That might sound like the result of a split personality but then when it comes to dieting it can often feel like we're in the situation where there's a devil on one shoulder and an angel on the other. One side is pulling you towards perfect attendance at the gym and a 100% paleo diet for the rest of your life. The other is reminding you that life is short and that lager is tasty.

If you feel like this, know that the answer lies between those two extremes. We aren't built to live at the extremes – it's great to have healthy ambitions but they have to be realistic – no one is perfect and if you stray you have to get used to forgiving yourself, by accepting what has happened, picking yourself up and getting back on with your journey. You won't get fit and healthy by listening to the angel, you'll get frustrated and tired. You won't get fat and unfit by listening to the devil on your shoulder every once in a while. Remember to balance those two extremes and keep being sympathetic to yourself – the biggest damage you can do to any diet is turning a slip-up into a decision to stop.

WHY DON'T OTHER PEOPLE SUPPORT YOU?

It can be frustrating and upsetting to feel that some of those people who are supposed to be on your side are actually thwarting your efforts to lose weight. Your friends, colleagues, family and partner – surely they have to help you out? But for nearly a third of men these are the people who put them off. What would cause them to do this?

THEY DON'T KNOW IT'S IMPORTANT TO YOU

Quite simply, do they know what this means to you? If you showed them your goals and told them about the life that you want to live and the things that you wanted to do, what would their reaction be? If the thought of telling them makes you feel embarrassed then perhaps you're not giving them the opportunity to be supportive, because why would they give you a boost up when perhaps they think that you're happy where you are? Equally, if you think that if you shared this dream with them then they would laugh then there are more serious problems with those relationships. Although a certain amount of mickey-taking is often a sign of a healthy relationship, it has its limits.

TIP   *Imagine telling people close to you about your goals – would they support you? If not, consider what that means about this relationship. If you can't consider talking to them about your goals, ask yourself why and what this means about where you are at this moment in time.*

THEY ARE JEALOUS YOU WANT TO CHANGE

This is quite a powerful reason that is tied to our identity and our roles within certain social groups. We can often fall into the habit of having set 'types' and find ourselves conforming to those roles, for no other reason than it's expected of us. If you are the "fat one" in your group then maybe it's accepted that you would finish off everyone else's dinner, or down your drink on a night out. For partners, especially those who live together, it can be hard to make progress when your significant other might not be in a place to accept your decision to change. From feelings of insecurity about their own health and weight they may find it easier to not support you, or to flatout sabotage your efforts.

TIP *Could the people who are jealous be enlisted into helping themselves change? If not, you will have to accept that these people – at least initially – are not going to be a source of support. Don't feel angry about that. Focus on your own goals and build a support network away from those people, but always allow that as you start to succeed they may want to catch up with you – which is where you can help to support them.*

THEY DON'T UNDERSTAND HOW THEY'RE NOT HELPING

You might live in a culture where the way that love is expressed is through plates groaning with food. Refusing the massed portions can be problematic because it's often perceived as pushing that love away. You might also get this from a partner who loves to bake, so you often find yourself surrounded by cakes. Perhaps the way that you traditionally socialise is through a night out at the pub or curry house and to break away from that would be seen as rejecting the friendship.

> **TIP** *Working around this means letting people know what you're trying to achieve. You have to explain what you are doing and why it matters to you, and get people excited about your challenge. You also have to be able to explain how you need things to change to help you reach your goals. The ones who listen will be converted into supporters and, at least for a short time, you need to replace the ones who don't support you with others who do.*

BUILDING YOUR SUPPORT TEAM

The idea of this preparation is to surround yourself with people and voices that know what you want to do and are cheering you on. We all know that sports teams gain a huge boost from playing at home because they are surrounded by faces and voices that are encouraging them and want to see them do well. This is what you are now going to build up.

Let's return to those five people who you spend the most time with. It's time to approach them with your goals. You can do this in any way you feel most comfortable – a face-to-face chat, an email or a phone call. The important thing is that this makes these people aware of what you are going to do.

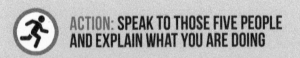

ACTION: SPEAK TO THOSE FIVE PEOPLE AND EXPLAIN WHAT YOU ARE DOING

Tell them what you will have to change to reach your goals and explain how this might change your behaviour in the coming months. Ask them if they can support you during this time. If it makes it easier, consider phrasing this as a challenge or a bet and encourage them to get involved. Note their responses and accept that if they cannot support you then you will need to find support in other places.

RECRUITING MORE SUPPORTERS

Where can you find other supporters for your weight loss? Everywhere! Here are some starting points. Don't feel that you have to limit yourself – it's better to have more support than you need.

ONLINE
MAN V FAT

Join **www.manvfat.com** for free and you will be joining the world's largest weight-loss community exclusively for men. You can get assistance in the Talk forums, find other men doing the same diet as you, join in challenges, log your weight at weekly or monthly weigh-ins, read blog posts and articles on a number of weight-loss issues and enter competitions.

SOCIAL NETWORKS

If you use Reddit, Facebook, Twitter or Instagram then there are thousands of pages out there that can give you doses of inspiration and support for free at any time of the day or night. As your timeline fills up with posts detailing challenges and motivational pictures, it can be really encouraging to see this sort of thing on a daily basis.

WEBSITES

If you're looking for some good sources of motivation then check out **www. manvfat.com/resources** where you'll find some of the best links to diet inspiration on the web.

BLOGGERS

Following other men's weight-loss blogs can give you an insight into dieting tips and training advice, while it can also be rewarding to see how other men are coping with the same challenges you are going through. Find our favourites on **www.manvfat.com/resources**.

OFFLINE
A PROFESSIONAL

Whether it's a dietician, a personal trainer or a member of the gym staff – if you have someone you have to look in the eyes on a regular basis then you will be more likely to be kept tuned into your weight loss.

WEIGHT-LOSS GROUPS

If your chosen diet has a support group element, could you attend? It may be that it is more focused on women, but that doesn't mean that you won't be welcomed, or that you can't use them as a support. The group leader should be a fount of knowledge about your diet and will have worked through the common problems you are likely to experience on a number of occasions.

WORK

Could you start a weight-loss group at your office? This could be done in the form of a bet to lose x% of your bodyweight (although try to keep timescales out of the bet itself). This is useful because it's a form of competition that you can't escape from which makes it a constant source of motivation.

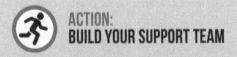

ACTION:
BUILD YOUR SUPPORT TEAM

Using the various sources above – go and recruit your support team. Go for a mix of on- and off-line partners. Find the ones who really believe in you and will cheer you on. Finding people who offer good encouragement can really make the difference between success and failure. Build your weight-loss team and fill it with people who motivate you.

TRACKING AND REVIEWING YOUR PROGRESS

Tracking is the single most essential tool in weight loss. By tracking your progress you hold yourself accountable to your aims, you plot and witness your journey towards your goals, while by reviewing your progress you learn about what is working and, more importantly, what isn't. Even if the diet you are following doesn't call for a log to be kept then you should still consider it essential. Knowing what you've eaten, what exercise you've done and keeping in touch with your progress towards your goals is the heart and soul of weight loss.

WHY TRACK?

The process of tracking your weight loss has two purposes. On one level the process of seeing what progress you're making can be incredibly motivational. There's nothing like seeing the numbers on the scale dropping and realising that your diet is actually working. It's only by giving yourself as complete a picture as possible that you can hope to see that. The very act of tracking is often enough to make you aware of the shortcuts you know you're taking but have previously chosen to ignore.

The other reason that tracking is so essential is because when progress slows, stops or reverses then the only resource you have to understand why is your tracking information. If you can look back over the last couple of weeks and identify what's going wrong, then you are still on course. By tracking you will also have a blueprint of those weeks that worked really well, which means you can replicate them for future success. You can also use it to reach out to your support network and get their input. If you haven't tracked then you would have to rely on your memories, which might be vague at best, or simply wrong.

TIP *The process of finding the best lifestyle for you is an ongoing investigation which will require a lot of learning and changing. You WILL have to adapt the way you've always done things. Ultimately, flexibility of thinking will be a key part of your success.*

The key to tracking and reviewing is to set up a reasonable system that works for you. An ideal system is laid out below.

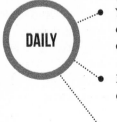

Your activity – what obligatory and optional activity you did over the course of the day, how it felt and any times, scores or distances you want to record.

Everything you are eating and drinking (including condiments, drinks, food stolen off other's plates).

How you're feeling – how your health is (illnesses, injury niggles), your struggles, successes, anything you've learned, questions you want to research the answers to.

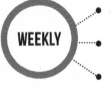

Weight – see opposite for details on how to track.

Fitness – how you are doing in relationship to your goals.

Off-the-scale victories (compliments, clothes fitting better, fitness achievements, etc).

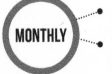

Body measurements.

Pictures – it's your choice whether you want to take a full body shot with complete side and front views, or if you'd just prefer a snapshot of your gut. Whichever it is, try not to accidentally upload it to Facebook.

HOW TO TRACK

There are two main ways to track your activity and eating. The first is to find a notebook or a page-a-day diary that you can keep next to your bed. In this you can spend the last five minutes of the day writing down what you've eaten, along with your activity and any of the tracking measurements that you're recording. It might seem strange at first to be recording this information but it will build up into an incredibly useful resource.

PROS
- Doesn't run out of batteries
- Can be organised however you want

CONS
- Not 'smart' – won't tell you how many calories your lunch was
- Doesn't allow you to network with other people

The second option is to use a tracking app. Most of these apps work on a variety of smartphone platforms and are free to use.

PROS
- Smarter
- Brings accountability to your tracking – other people can see what you've tracked and whether you've hit your goals

CONS
- Takes longer than writing in a diary
- Stuck with the format that the app maker uses
- Possible charges in the future

HOW TO TRACK YOUR WEIGHT

As seen in the equipment section, it's vital that you choose a quality set of scales that can be relied upon to give you accurate results.

When you weigh yourself is a personal decision – some people weigh themselves daily, some weekly, fortnightly or monthly. You want to choose a weigh-in frequency that gives you a picture of your general weight loss without confusing or demotivating you. Sometimes with a weekly weigh-in you can find that you've had a brilliant week with eating and activity but you've actually put on weight. Your weight will fluctuate hugely depending on a number of issues:

- How hydrated you are
- When you weigh yourself
- What you're wearing
- Where the scales are placed (hard floor or carpet)
- Bowel movements

 TIP *Don't forget that a good week on the diet might not translate into a weight loss until the following week.*

Personally, I know that a fortnightly or a monthly weigh-in would be better for me and give me a clearer idea of my overall weight trends, but I can't resist a weekly weigh-in. To weigh properly make sure you do the following:

- Weigh first thing in the morning
- Weigh naked
- Weigh after using the toilet
- Place the scales in exactly the same place on the bathroom floor

REVIEWING

Tracking is all about gathering the information, reviewing is about sifting through the information you have collected, pulling out insights and deciding on changes to your diet.

WHY MONTHLY?

Let's take the example of weight loss. You need a month's worth of information to have any valid insight. If you reviewed your diet after a week based on one weigh-in then you might well find that you come to a false conclusion.

HOW TO REVIEW

Make no mistake about it – this is the most valuable and important research project

'If things are not going well, then this is the point that you can start to understand why. Refresh yourself on your diet's principles, compare these to your tracking information and see where you've deviated from them. Go to your supporters and ask them to look through your tracking data and see if they can understand what's happening. Make sure that you are selective about what advice you take, though. Don't just respond to the first, or the loudest, voice.'

you've ever done. Treat it with the seriousness it deserves and give it your full attention! Read through your tracking information. Look at your goals and see how you've made steps towards those goals. If you've earned a reward then claim it! Be honest – lying to yourself will simply cause frustration and failure.

If things are not going well, then this is the point where you can start to understand why. Refresh yourself on your diet's principles, compare these to your tracking information and see where you've deviated from them. Go to your supporters and ask them to look through your tracking data and see if they can understand what's happening. Make sure that you are selective about what advice you take, though. Don't just respond to the first, or the loudest, voice.

At your review you might like to select a new habit to add into your existing weight loss. Perhaps you'd like to start experimenting with adding probiotics to your diet and seeing what impact they have. Track one change at a time. As well as keeping your schedule achievable it also means that you will have a better chance of seeing what difference that one change makes – alter more than one variable at the same time and it will be very difficult to know precisely what made a difference.

DAILY TRACKING SHEET

MONDAY		
Food and drink	**Activity**	**How you're feeling**

TUESDAY		
Food and drink	**Activity**	**How you're feeling**

WEDNESDAY		
Food and drink	**Activity**	**How you're feeling**

THURSDAY		
Food and drink	**Activity**	**How you're feeling**

FRIDAY

Food and drink	Activity	How you're feeling

SATURDAY

Food and drink	Activity	How you're feeling

SUNDAY

Food and drink	Activity	How you're feeling

RESEARCH AND REVIEW

Questions, problems, ideas, lessons learned

WEEKLY TRACKING SHEET

WEEK 1

Weight	Fitness	Off the scales	Measurements	Goals hit

WEEK 2

Weight	Fitness	Off the scales	Measurements	Goals hit

WEEK 3

Weight	Fitness	Off the scales	Measurements	Goals hit

WEEK 4

Weight	Fitness	Off the scales	Measurements	Goals hit

WEEK 5

Weight	Fitness	Off the scales	Measurements	Goals hit

MAKING A DAY PLAN

It's comforting to know that what constitutes a perfect day will depend largely on what your preferences are. Running a marathon might make some dance with joy, but the thought could send others sobbing to their bed. This perfect day plan might not fit your routine, but it should give you an idea of how to fit some of the key considerations into your routine.

- Attend to your digestion
- Eat within your nutritional choices
- Tracking
- Hydration
- Exercise
- Fun!
- Sleep

SAMPLE PLAN FOR A 'PERFECT' DAY

06.30 WAKING

Try a natural light alarm clock if you suffer from irritability first thing in the morning. Time to get your head straight. Meditate, refresh your motivational thoughts, reflect. Drink at least a pint of filtered water to get your system going.

06.45–07.30 EXERCISE

Start with some stretching and flexibility work then cardio. Rehydrate after exercise.

07.30–07.45 WASHING/DRESSING

Try switching to cold at the end of the shower to boost testosterone production, improve circulation and wake yourself up!

07.45–08.20 BREAKFAST AND SUPPLEMENTS

Start with kefir (see page 236) to give your gut a good start to the day. Take any supplements and vitamins you are currently trialling. Take on plenty of fluids during breakfast.

08.20–09.00 COMMUTE TO WORK

Head to work by bike, walking, running or using the train/bus and walking for the last few stops.

09.00 WORK

While you're at work set an alarm so that every 50 minutes you take a break and do something that requires you to move – whether that's moving around the building, going outside for some fresh air or simply using a standing desk. Schedule walking meetings to avoid chair time, stand when you're on the phone and always use the stairs. Keep water with you and refill regularly. Stick to water or herbal teas.

10.30 SNACK

12.30–13.30 LUNCH HOUR

During your lunch hour make sure you get up and move around, even if you just walk to the shop to get your lunch. Eating al desko is never a good idea. Ideally, see if you can get out of your workplace altogether as a break both for your mind and for your body. Lunch should be a bigger meal than the evening meal so that your body has time to digest. Hydrate. If you didn't get to exercise earlier then take the time to get out for a run, a cycle, swim or simply a long walk around the building.

15.30 SNACK

18.00
COMMUTE HOME

As for the morning journey, make sure that you incorporate some form of movement into your commute.

18.30 DINNER
Eat early with plenty of water to maximise your gut health and give yourself plenty of time to digest.

19.00 AFTER-DINNER WALK
A great way to improve your digestion and fit in some more calorie expenditure.

19.30–22.30 PREPARE
Prepare tomorrow's lunch, batch cook some foods, relax, socialise, research new healthy habits you want to make.

21.30 ELECTRONICS OFF
Switch off for at least an hour before bedtime to maximise melatonin production and prepare yourself for sleep.

22.25–22.30 TRACKING
Fill in your tracking for the day's nutrition and activity.

22.30 SLEEPING
Sleep in a completely dark bedroom, free from noise and light sources. Practise meditation before you sleep and try a valerian or camomile tea and lavender essential oils to aid a restful night's sleep.

MAKING A WEEK PLAN

As with the perfect day plan this might not work exactly with your lifestyle but it gives you a sample plan of how a week can work out and how you can balance all of the things that you have to address.

The elements to include on a weekly basis:

- Planning – plan your meals on a weekly basis. On your calendar you should identify times when your motivation will be challenged and plan how you'll cope with those times
- Shopping – monthly food delivery, weekly fruit and veg shop, visit the butchers once a week
- Measurements (tracking)
- Plan and diarise sessions of exercise to ensure they don't get forgotten. Identify times during the week when you could up your obligatory activity – could you walk or cycle to events, or change arrangements to take a healthier option?
- Organisation – cleaning, cooking and other errands
- Work – have a forward view of what is going on with work (trips away, special events, busy periods) and plan and prepare for how this might affect your health – schedule relaxation or meditation around particularly busy times
- Vitamins and supplements topped up and portioned out for the following week (consider getting a pill box to help plan this)

SAMPLE PLAN FOR THE 'PERFECT' WEEK

SUN

- Cleaning house
- Cooking in batches for week ahead
- Early night for a good start to week
- Rest day – every week you should have at least one rest day where you allow the body to fully recover. If you can schedule a relaxation therapy such as massage or reflexology then do so

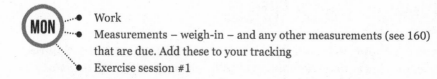
MON
- Work
- Measurements – weigh-in – and any other measurements (see 160) that are due. Add these to your tracking
- Exercise session #1

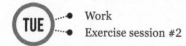
TUE
- Work
- Exercise session #2

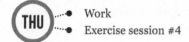
WED
- Work
- Exercise session #3 or Rest day

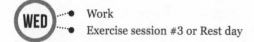
THU
- Work
- Exercise session #4

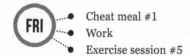
FRI
- Cheat meal #1
- Work
- Exercise session #5

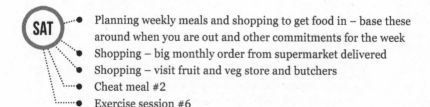
SAT
- Planning weekly meals and shopping to get food in – base these around when you are out and other commitments for the week
- Shopping – big monthly order from supermarket delivered
- Shopping – visit fruit and veg store and butchers
- Cheat meal #2
- Exercise session #6

CHANGING YOUR MINDSET

You are about to commit to a new, healthier lifestyle and that requires a moment of serious thought. After all, beating fat is going to make a huge difference to your life. Therefore taking five minutes to change your mindset is the perfect final step before you get going.

1. SAY GOODBYE TO THE FAT YOU

You've made your preparations, you understand what you're doing and you're ready to get on with it. It's essential that you take the time to say goodbye to 'fat you'. This is a process that can take time so don't worry if it's ongoing – the important thing is that you mentally say goodbye to the person you were and start to think, act and behave like the person you have decided to become. This means that your reactions, your feelings and your emotions can undergo a severe change – you start to think like healthy you. This is the filter that you use from now on – it's no longer the 'fat you' thinking that made you unhappy and that you so desperately want to change – but the new healthy you who wants good things for your body, your mind and your health.

It's vital that you take souvenirs. You might not think you will ever want them but get some high-resolution images of you before you started to lose the weight. Get a good camera and let it all hang out – a front and side picture in your underwear is usually enough. These photos are a vivid reminder of where you were and where you do not want to go back to. Frankly, they're also going to be used for boasting – a lot. You are the next MAN v FAT Amazing Loser. Don't forget you will not be coming back to this place again. Record the sensations in any way you choose. A video, photos, an entry in your tracking book about how it feels to be at this point – what it's like to shop for clothes at this size, how you feel when your partner or family look at you. Any comments that have been said to you about your weight.

Take a moment and enjoy saying goodbye to fat you.

2. SEE YOURSELF CROSSING THE FINISH LINE

The clearer you can see where you are going to be, the more effective your weight loss will be. You already have the black-and-white goals that you've stated earlier, but it's important to also build up a picture of how it will really feel when you end up reaching your goal.

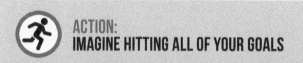 **ACTION:**
IMAGINE HITTING ALL OF YOUR GOALS

What will it feel like when you get there? How will people react and what sort of things will you hear them say? Record these feelings. When you reach your goal, what will life be like for you? How will it change the way you think and move? How will it change what you do? If you struggle to imagine it, then consider asking other people who have lost weight. Read the stories of the Amazing Losers and borrow the way that they felt.

Record in as much detail as possible how you imagine it feels at your finish line:

_____

_____

_____

_____

'Listen out for the positive words that you imagine people using about you. Be on the alert for all of those good feelings that you anticipate feeling. Understand that your goals are going to happen – your mind already knows it, your body just has to catch up.'

As you build up a detailed picture of what you are going to be like in the future, start to notice these things happening as you lose weight. Listen out for the positive words that you imagine people using about you. Be on the alert for all of those good feelings that you anticipate feeling. Understand that your goals are going to happen – your mind already knows it, your body just has to catch up.

3. ENJOY IT

Finally – at this very moment – let go of any fear, anger or resentment towards what you are doing. You have no need to be scared – your tracking and reviewing will ensure that any bumps in the road will soon get dealt with. You have chosen your diet well, you know what you're doing and you know that you have a team of supporters who cannot wait to see you succeed. You understand that your activity levels are going to change, but that they're changing into something that you can do, and into things you want to do. You are about to gain so much that your life will be full in ways that you hadn't even anticipated. You are going to lose weight, but you are going to gain life.

Let's get started.

THE FINAL CHECKLIST — READY TO GO?

- [ ] Have you signed up with **www.manvfat.com?**

- [ ] Do you understand what made you fat in the first place?

- [ ] Have you taken steps to address those issues?

- [ ] Have you understood what calories are and why they're important?

- [ ] Do you know the basics of nutrition?

- [ ] Have you chosen a diet plan to follow?

- [ ] Have you worked out where you can improve your obligatory activity?

- [ ] Are you ready to get going with optional activity again?

- [ ] Have you set out your goals and rewards?

- [ ] Have you got everything you need to do your diet?

- [ ] Have you identified any threats and assembled your support team?

- [ ] Do you know how you are tracking and reviewing?

- [ ] Have you said goodbye to fat you?

STEPHEN MORRISON

Age: 41 **Job:** Civil servant and physical activity champion
Height: 5' 9" (175.3cm) **Heaviest weight:** 334lb (151.5kg)
Lowest weight: 178lb (80.7kg)

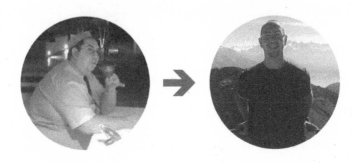

My change started when I saw a photo of myself. I looked in the mirror every day and I knew that I was morbidly obese, but until I saw that photo it didn't really dawn on me. In the photo I saw a look of fake happiness on my face. I realised that, although I was smiling in that picture, I was far from happy. I realised that I was lying to myself about my weight; that I was lying to everybody that I didn't care about it. It just shocked me to the core. From that moment on, I was relentless.

As a child I had Perthes Disease. It kept me confined to a wheelchair and on crutches and I had to go to a special needs school. I was told by a doctor that I'd never be as active as other children and that I would have lifelong problems with mobility. That mind-set just sunk in and I didn't test the truth of it until decades later. The thing that saved me from getting fat earlier was that I was in a job where I was on my feet most of the day. However, when I was 28, I settled down, got married and moved into a desk job in the civil service. The weight just piled on.

Most of my life I had yo-yo dieted and I realised that if I was going to be successful I couldn't repeat the mistakes of the past, that I would have to find out what more I could do. In my job I am a Lean Practitioner – it's a process management role that looks at systems and identifies root causes and solutions. I decided to apply this process to my life and asked myself what the problem was. The answer: I didn't move enough and ate too much. The other problem: I was unhappy and tracing it back, the root cause of it all was my obesity.

I didn't launch into an impossible-to-follow diet, I learned about what was causing me problems and I researched solutions. I thought, I'm not going to be crazy, I'm going to plan and prepare and work out how I'll take those steps to get me more active. I made meal plans, food lists and I planned my walks. After two weeks of planning, I was in a better place and confident. I had designed my own spreadsheet, where I added my daily activity and my intake, including the nutritional breakdown of every meal. Everything was evaluated daily to identify patterns.

At work, I told everyone I was losing weight and that I was going to be an Ironman and a marathon runner! 95% of the people I told laughed. I'd probably been saying this sort of thing for years, but I decided to make myself accountable, so every week I posted on the staff noticeboard how I'd done on my weigh-in that week. That was a big motivator when it came to the weekend and I was thinking of stuffing my face! Having prepared properly, the weight dropped off. At first, I was losing 10–12lb (4.5–5.5kg) a week which then dropped to 7 or 8lb. I lost 140lb (64kg) in 9 months.

There is a lot you can do to make yourself healthier and happier but it is all individual. There is no point telling me a cucumber is full of nutrients and vitamins – I still can't stand them. It's about making changes that you can actually sustain. There is no point telling someone they are going to run a marathon when putting on a pair of trainers scares them – take small steps, make small changes. On a practical level I'd say start sleeping more, start drinking more water, start asking yourself: 'Do I really want this food?' Accept that you will have a few failures but don't use those slips as an excuse to give up.

I'm now a marathon runner, a Lay Adviser to the Faculty of Sports and Exercise Medicine and a Fit in 14 Ambassador for the Scottish Government, while I am training to qualify as a personal trainer and coordinate Great Run Local in Glasgow. Nobody laughs at my goals now!
www.manvfat.com/members/stephen-morrison-779

SURYAGNI ROY

Age: 22 **Job:** Final year student **Height:** 5'10" (177.8cm)
Heaviest weight: 339.5lb (154kg) **Lowest weight:** 200.6lb (91kg)

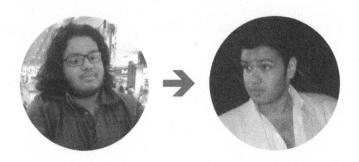

When I was big I was miserable. Honestly, life was tough. I can sum it up by saying that being fat isn't a crime, but I live in Calcutta which is a very busy and densely populated city and I have a lot of experience of being a big man in that city. You are just constantly aware of how much space you take up! Bumping into other people, feeling guilty when you ride on a bus or train – all of these things make the experience of being big miserable.

I started gaining weight at a frightening rate when I was around nine or 10 years of age. I remember this was a time when fast food restaurants like McDonald's and KFC began to appear in the city. I started to eat more burgers and chips and fried foods. I was eating them regularly, perhaps three or more times per week, and the weight started to pile on quickly. The worst thing for me though was the arrival in my life of Pepsi! Every day I would drink a litre or two, which without me really thinking about it was giving me around 1,000 extra calories before I even started to eat any food! Because I wasn't really eating sweets or crisps, I thought I had quite a healthy diet – the weight gain was a mystery to me and I chose not to see it.

The final issue that led to me gaining weight was skipping breakfast, which I see now was just a horrific mistake. I was always too busy to eat in the mornings and never really felt hungry so I would just leave the house with no food. Again, I think it made me feel like I was a healthier person. But I see now that it led to low blood sugar and over-eating at other parts of the day – it also led me to make bad decisions about getting food when I was out because I was starving. Add into this the fact that I wasn't active at all and you have a recipe for disaster!

I had to change because all my life I have wanted to be an actor. In my heart I knew that the opportunities I would get at my largest were not good. Take one look on TV and in films and tell me how many fat leading actors you see? The answer is none. I believe that in life if you want to achieve something great then it starts with you. For me, the realisation was that it was in my power to lose weight and create the life I wanted for myself.

In addition to this I am very blessed to be close to my family. I have a wonderful mother, father, kid brother and friends. They were all my inspiration and supporters. My little brother is an active cricketer and he is the captain for the school team. Looking at him I felt that I wasn't providing the sort of role model that an older brother should – I wanted to be someone that he could look up to and respect. I did not feel like that person at 339lb (154kg). So this was the point that I decided to look at my life and make a positive change.

I changed my diet so that I was eating more protein and cut out the Pepsi. I also started using the gym. In the gym I alternated my days so on one day I would do cardio and on the next I would focus on strength training. For me this meant that I got the best returns and the variety meant that I didn't get bored. If it's cardio then I would try and do running on the treadmill, or a variety of Crossfit exercises where there is cardio twinned with weights. So I might have been running with a heavy ball, or doing squats and jumps with weights. On strength days I would work with my trainers to learn good form and look to improve the weights I could lift, which would help me build muscle and drop fat. Weight lifting is excellent if you are looking to lose weight, it might not seem like it, but trust me, it works!
www.manvfat.com/members/suryagniroy

TROUBLESHOOTING

If you're experiencing a problem with any aspect of your weight loss then this is the place to pin it down, work out what's going wrong and take the steps to solve it.

PROBLEM	CAUSE
I'm starving!	• Not eating enough! • Not eating the right foods
I spend my life craving chocolate/beer/ crisps/carbs/etc	• This is the psychological impact of saying that you absolutely can't have that thing – it's all your mind thinks about and you end up craving it
I keep changing my mind about what diet to do	• Not enough research meaning you don't pick the right diet for you • Listening to every opinion going on diet • Motivation not strong enough at this time

SOLUTION
• Urgently check whether your daily calorie intake is meeting your calorie needs (see page 61). If not then you need to address this, or risk doing yourself serious damage. • Try hydrating properly and bulking up the quantity of your meals with low-calorie, nutritionally dense foods like vegetables. • Make sure you are getting a portion of protein with each meal to ensure you feel full. • Consider switching to a diet that allows for unlimited foods (but be mindful that the calorie limits still apply). See page 67. • Make sure you build in regular snacks to keep your blood sugar levels even throughout the day. • Follow mindful eating techniques to increase your awareness of what you are currently eating. See page 138.
• Switch to a diet that allows for any foods, such as a calorie-controlled diet. See page 73. • Think about introducing a cheat meal/day where you can indulge in these items. See page 136.
• Do some proper research about which diet will fit best with your lifestyle. When you have chosen a diet, research how you will fit it into your life. • Start to be more selective about who you listen to about weight loss. • Return to your motivation exercise (see page 31) and create a real and vivid picture of how you want your life to be.

PROBLEM	CAUSE
I can't eat breakfast	• Many men feel that breakfast is too early to start eating • Some actually feel nauseous in the morning
It's Christmas / a music festival / my birthday / my third cousin's 7th wedding anniversary	• A rare time to party has presented itself and you don't want to miss out
I'm injured	• Almost all injuries are related to trying to do too much too quickly, or a trip, slip or over-enthusiastic tackle from your best mate
I've hit a plateau	• Weight loss hasn't dropped for weeks/months
My partner/ friend/ mum doesn't support me	• Jealousy • Not understanding why this is important to you • Not understanding how they're damaging your efforts

SOLUTION
<ul><li>Consider using Intermittent Fasting (see page 140) as a way of fitting a sensible calorie intake into a day, without forcing you to eat early.</li><li>Equally, if you feel that you can drink in the morning, then consider a liquid breakfast of a juice, protein shake or smoothie.</li></ul>
<ul><li>Save up for it – make sure you're particularly good on your diet and with your exercise before the event you're excited about and then go for it. Treat it as your cheat meal and then focus on getting straight back on track afterwards.</li><li>Go to the event but eat before you get there and focus more on the people and the dancing (great cardio) than the food and drink. 'We don't have to take our clothes off to have a good time,' explained Jermaine Stewart and he was right – but did you know that the original lyric was 'We don't have to spend all day eating carbs and getting leathered to have a good time'? The man really knew his stuff.</li></ul>
<ul><li>See a professional – your doctor should be able to diagnose and refer you to an appropriate specialist. Failure to do this will simply result in the injury taking longer to heal, or possibly leave you with lasting damage.</li></ul>
<ul><li>Check you're tracking everything and not straying from the rules of the diet you're following.</li><li>If you're content that you're eating at a deficit, then try completely changing your activity for at least two weeks. Pick something different you fancy trying and switch it up. Often this is enough to move things along.</li><li>Have patience. You didn't get fat overnight and the weight will take time to come off. Forget about the numbers on the scales and focus instead on your fitness goals and whether you are getting closer to those.</li><li>DO NOT get frustrated and give in. Everyone experiences these stages of a diet.</li></ul>
See page 176.

PROBLEM	CAUSE
I have a cold/flu/ illness	• Bacteria/germs/pushing your body too hard with exercise
I'm good during the week, awful at the weekend	• Choosing too strict a diet can leave you feeling that you need to go really wild at the weekend. • Motivation is weak.
I'm getting bored of eating the same thing over and over again	• A lack of preparation leads to you sticking to your diet by eating the same thing over and over again.
I'm too tired to diet	• Lack of proper sleep • Medical condition • Poor nutrition • Stress

SOLUTION

- It's normal to pick up the occasional short-term illness, but it's worth addressing the state of your immune system.
- Being ill disrupts weight loss, so don't expect to see a big change on the scales.
- Keep focused on your diet and especially emphasise making sure you're getting enough fruit and vegetables to support your body.
- Scale back your exercise plans while you're feeling ill. You are the best judge of whether you're well enough to exercise; in some cases it can speed up your recovery but in others it can seriously threaten your health.

- Research different diets and pick one that seems to give you a better balance for your life – whether that's choosing one that allows you to have a couple of glasses of wine every day or one that gives you an 'allowance' you can spend however you like.
- Consider adding a cheat meal/day to your weight loss and experiment with whether you can still lose weight in that way.
- Address your motivation issues – see page 30.

- Research. Take the time to learn about your diet and to understand what you can and can't have.
- Motivation – revisit your motivation and ask whether you are committed to a healthy programme of weight loss. If not, get back and supercharge your motivation. See page 31.
- Planning – a good daily and weekly plan can ensure that you've got enough time to think in advance about what you're eating and gives you the opportunity to prepare a whole range of foods that you enjoy and that fit in with your diet.
- Activate your support network. Check online and ask people for help.

- Address the various issues that result in fatigue.
- Understand that getting a healthy and balanced diet (one that contains foods from all the major food groups) is the ideal way to fuel your body, give you energy and make you feel less tired.
- Examine your motivation – see page 30.

PROBLEM	CAUSE
I hate vegetables	• Personal preference • Lack of exposure to good sources of vegetables and different ways of preparing them
I'm following the diet but I just can't lose weight!	• Undeclared, subconscious consuming • Not being honest with yourself • Over-calculating the amount of calories removed by exercise • Medical issue
I'm embarrassed at the gym	• Unfriendly gym goers • Unsure of what exercise to be doing for the best returns • Not sure what to wear

SOLUTION

- You will be healthier if you eat a balanced diet, including large portions of vegetables and fruits, so try to learn to love them.
- If there are a couple of vegetables you like, simply stick to those.
- Experiment with new vegetables and different ways of cooking them – boiled cauliflower is unrecognisable from spiced and roasted cauliflower.
- Spend more on organic fresh vegetables and fruits – the bags of frozen veg are a pale, frosty imitation of the real thing.
- Blitz your fruit and veg into sauces and smoothies and pretend they're not actually there.

- First return to the plan and make sure that you are actually creating a deficit in your calories. Try weighing everything for a few days to make sure that you are not accidentally taking more from a bigger portion or adding hundreds of extra calories with sauces and oils.
- Ensure you count everything from the small bits of food you steal off other people's plates, to sauces and travel sweets – EVERYTHING!
- Keep exercising but try not counting the calories for the exercise you have been doing.
- Follow this plan for a fortnight at least and then weigh yourself.
- If you are still in the same position then check a range of measurements – it could be that you are gaining muscle mass while losing fat.
- Check you are weighing yourself correctly on an accurate pair of scales.
- Speak to your doctor about your concerns and ask for a range of tests that could determine if there is a health issue.

- Find a better gym, or forget the gym! If you hate other people watching you on a treadmill, go for a run in a quiet wood.
- Do some research and experiment at home to give you confidence before you hit the gym – try following the Bodyweight Strength Fitness Plan on page 120.
- Do some research about what people are wearing and treat yourself to some new clothes when you hit a weight-loss target.

PROBLEM	CAUSE
I'm getting a lot of loose skin	• When you gain weight your skin stretches to accommodate your growth • When you lose weight the elasticity of the skin takes time to shrink back – this results in loose skin
I think I've gone into starvation mode	• Belief that lowering your calorie intake slows down your metabolism and makes it harder or impossible for you to lose weight
I've lost weight but I'm still unhappy	• Other sources of unhappiness in your life

SOLUTION
<ul><li>If you have a lot of weight to lose then your skin may take time to regain its elasticity and shrink back down to your size. Be patient.</li><li>Consider surgery to remove the loose skin.</li><li>Make sure you are very well hydrated – your skin's elasticity depends largely on the level of hydration in your body.</li><li>Lose weight at a sensible rate – if you drop weight very quickly then it's more likely that you will end up with loose skin.</li><li>Improve your muscle tone with exercise and activity.</li></ul>
<ul><li>Check you are following your diet properly. If you are then you will lose weight – it's as simple as that.</li><li>Stop weighing yourself so regularly. Focus on your other goals for a month or two before weighing yourself again.</li><li>Relax – although starvation mode is discussed a lot it's a concept that's almost entirely irrelevant to your situation.</li></ul>
<ul><li>Don't assume that losing weight will fix everything such as damaged relationships, make you love a terrible job, cure your halitosis, etc.</li><li>Losing weight will make you more confident but that in itself might expose other problems.</li><li>Losing weight can actually put pressure on relationships – especially if one party feels like they're being 'left behind'.</li><li>See the sections on Building Your Support Team and Identifying Threats – pages 176–182.</li></ul>

GLOSSARY OF JARGON

Blood Glucose/Blood Sugar – the levels of glucose found in the blood. Glucose from the liver and intestines is carried to cells around the body by the bloodstream, where the hormone insulin makes it available for absorption by the cells.

Calorie – a unit of energy which is stated as the amount of energy needed to raise the temperature of one gramme of water by one degree Celsius. The calorie is widely used as the main measurement of food energy.

Carboyhdrates – are chains of sugars that the body has to break down to use as energy. Simple (or fast) carbohydrates are those that are quick to break down and mean that the body can very quickly access them as a source of energy. Complex (or slow) carbs are those foods that the digestive system requires more time to access, thus keeping you fuller for longer. To see whether a carbohydrate is fast or slow simply look at its Glycaemic Index score.

CHD – Coronary Heart Disease.

Cheat Meal – a weight-loss technique where you suspend the normal rules of your diet. This is normally done either for a single meal or an entire day. During this period many men take the opportunity to consume the things that they might be missing on the 'normal' days of their diet.

CICO – abbreviation of Calories In Calories Out, sometimes also known as the energy balance – the amount of energy you take in, compared to the amount you expend.

Cortisol – the 'stress' hormone. Cortisol is released in response to fear or attack by the adrenal glands. High cortisol levels lower your ability to learn, impair your immune system and increase weight gain.

Fat – a macronutrient used as a form of energy by the body with an energy value of 9 calories per gramme (see also carbohydrates and protein).Tthere are three types of fats: saturated, unsaturated and trans fats. Saturated fats are found in animal products and processed foods. Unsaturated fats come from plant sources such as oil from nuts, avocados and olives. Trans fats are almost exclusively made in a laboratory by adding hydrogen to vegetable oils.

Gastric Band – an example of bariatric surgery, a gastric band (also called a lap band or a LAGB) is a band that is fitted around the top of the stomach. This reduces the volume of food that can be eaten and also means food needs to be eaten slower, which reduces the calories that a person can consume and results in weight loss. There are several huge drawbacks to gastric band surgery – not least the 1 in 1000 chance of death.

Gluten – a mixture of two proteins found in grains – especially wheat.

Glycaemic Index (GI) – a measurement of how quickly a food can be broken down to elevate the blood sugar.

IIFYM – If It Fits Your Macros (see Macros).

Insulin – hormone produced by the pancreas responsible for the absorption of glucose into the body's cells.

Ketosis – when the body stops breaking down carbohydrates for energy and starts to break down fat. This process produces ketones which are detectable in the blood, urine and sometimes on the breath.

Legumes – plants, but it's usually the fruit or seeds of those plants. Think of foods that originally grow in a pod – such as peas, lentils and beans.

Light (or 'Lite') – a food label that requires the product to be 30% lower in one value (such as calories or fat) than the ordinary version of the product.

Low fat – a food product that either has naturally low levels of fat or one that has been altered to reduce the amount of fat it contains. Typically, products that are lower than 3 grammes of fat per 100 grammes are allowed to be described as low fat.

Macros – macronutrients, the main groups of nutrients that the body needs to be healthy. The three main macros are protein, fat and carbohydrates.

Metabolism – a catch-all term for the chemical reactions that happen in the cells of our bodies to keep us alive.

No Added Sugar – a food label that simply means no additional sugar has been added. This does not mean that there is no sugar in it.

Protein – a macronutrient group built from amino acids. There are 22 amino acids that are essential to humans, nine of which we need to get exclusively from food.

Satiety Index – a means of rating which foods are most likely to keep you feeling fuller for longer. White bread is the base measure and foods that score higher than 100 are said to be more filling than white bread, a score of less than 100 means they are less filling than white bread. High SI foods are full of proteins and fibre.

VLCD – Very Low Calorie Diet – anything where you would regularly consume under 800 calories per day, although this definition varies. VLCDs should only be undertaken after a medical consultation.

TIM BAUER

Age: 34 **Job:** Marketing director **Height:** 6'4" (193cm)
Heaviest weight: 440lb (199.6kg) **Lowest weight:** 211lb (95.7kg)

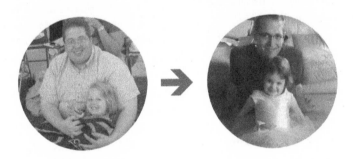

Growing up, my parents were both in food service so we ate very well. I was mostly raised in restaurants and, as a kid, when we went out to eat I could order whatever I wanted – and kids don't order quinoa! So I'd eat pasta with macaroni and cheese on the side, the bread bowls would always be refilled and we ate like kings. I wasn't a depressed kid but whenever I had problems I would go to the fridge and there was always ice cream, pasta, big portions of heavy food. When I got married at 21 it got even worse. I just basically let myself go and gained another 80lb (36kg). I was already 360lb (163kg) and I went up to 440lbs (199kg).

One day I was preparing a lesson for a church class that was talking about how to handle your challenges. The way I was teaching it was where you used tennis balls and wrote names of different sins on them and you'd throw the balls to the kids at the same time and obviously they couldn't catch them all. But when these things came at them one at a time they could deal with them all individually. It listed a load of different sins to write on the balls and alongside adultery, dishonesty and murder was unhealthy eating habits. I was thinking about my two little girls and as I read it I thought I'm breaking oaths against God and setting a bad example for my kids. Something about that moment just struck me.

When I decided to make a change I didn't understand nutrition at all, so I started by following some diet plans a friend had given me but then I discovered paleo eating. Paleo gave me a healthy way to eat and a system to view food through. With paleo you eat like cavemen used to eat, it is a wholefoods-based diet that mostly abstains from three categories of food – grains, legumes and dairy. Most of my diet consists of meat and vegetables.

A lot of people on paleo follow this 80/20 rule where they'll let themselves go 20% of the time. I'm personally not the kind of person who can have cheat meals! For me, cheat meals turn into cheat days and cheat days turn into cheat weeks. So since November 2010 I have not had a single sugary dessert, not even a bit – if somebody says 'have a bit of a cupcake' then I say no. I could probably now have a bite of cake without ending up in the foetal position covered in whipped cream and sugar, but that being said I don't miss it – I don't want it – people say don't you miss ice cream? I just don't, I don't want it.

I thought losing weight would solve all my problems. I thought I would get healthy and everything would be cool, maybe my wife will love me more, maybe I would love myself more. So I got to the end of my rice-cake-and-treadmill-filled rainbow and there was no pot of gold there, everything wasn't perfect. So I decided OK, I lost weight, I dealt with my physical self, I am going to go into counselling and deal with those issues.

When I went to counselling and started dealing with my challenges what I found is that I have this need to be a perfect person, which obviously is an impossible goal and leads to disappointment. The way I would deal with that is I would turn to food to help myself and I was also punishing myself for being imperfect with food. After I'd had counselling I re-examined some of my beliefs and found I was part of a church where I didn't believe in everything they were practising, so I moved to a church I know is consistent with my spiritual beliefs. Everything is different now! This weight loss was so transforming that it gave me the ability to examine the other parts of my life as well, and it all started with tennis balls!
www.manvfat.com/members/tiniertim

ANDREW SHANAHAN

Age: 37 **Job:** Editor at MAN v FAT **Height:** 5'9" (175.3cm)
Heaviest weight: 229lb (103.9kg) **Lowest weight:** 162lb (73.5kg)

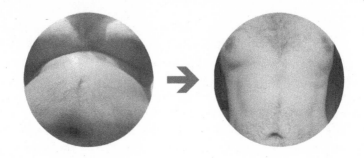

I've had weight problems in one way or another my entire life. When I was four my parents got divorced and we would spend every other weekend and some holidays with my dad and the rest of the time with my mum. I remember there being wildly different ways that food was consumed in each house. In my mum's house we ate a lot of vegetables because a lot of the food was grown on the allotment; when we went to my dad's it was big bags of sweets, rounds of toast and butter and enough arctic roll to bring down a polar bear. That period wrote the rules in my head about food. It was feast then famine. Binge then purge. Also it keyed into my mind that when you feel a bit sad then food can be a comfort.

A couple of years ago I was stressed with working on a project that required long hours and kept me immobile for long parts of the day. When I got home I'd reward myself with rubbish food and beer. One morning I was getting out of bed and I took a photo of my gut and chest. It was really horrific. Looking at the picture I knew I wanted to lose weight. I knew I had to change the way that I lived and fundamentally change the way I looked at food – I needed to beat the famine/feast cycle that I had as my blueprint for how to eat. I came up with some very simple rules that I resolved to follow.

1) Weigh and measure myself regularly and record what I ate

2) Eat much smaller portions of healthier foods
3) Get active
4) Have two cheat meals a week
5) Whenever I eat, ask myself if this food is helping me become who I want to be?

The last one was important because it caused me to confront a lot of the times when I ate not because I was hungry, but because I was stressed or angry. It made me see that I had problems like stress that were connected to me eating poorly, which had to be addressed if anything was going to change. I monitored my intake with a food diary and tracking on MyFitnessPal. What I quickly saw was that I was eating roughly the right things but I wasn't moving enough and I was eating gigantic portions.

I didn't consider myself to be dieting. I was just choosing to eat good stuff rather than wasteful calories. I think we all know what healthy food looks like, don't we? It looks like a balance. A balance of foods from different groups, including fats, carbs and a balance of colours. For breakfast I'd eat muesli with blueberries, lunch would be homemade soup, or a small chicken kebab and salad, and tea would be protein with vegetables and some carbs – maybe a beef stir fry with a small portion of noodles.

I made an appointment to see a local personal trainer and told him that I wanted him to build me up slowly over 10 weeks. It cost a fair amount but it's among the best money I've ever spent because it allowed me to get comfortable about exercising and being in an environment where I wasn't 100% sure I belonged. After 10 weeks of working with the trainer I felt like a different person. I was so much more confident. I'd started to explore other forms of fitness and realised that I absolutely loved yoga and even put in for my first triathlon. The key for me was taking it really slowly and working with someone I trusted. I also had someone shouting encouragement at me and I learned that that's a really powerful tool.

The best thing about losing weight is that for years I told myself I was one person and now I know I can change that definition. My advice if you want to lose weight is be brutally honest with yourself: if you're stressed – admit it and deal with it; if you need help – get it; if you're bored and eat a load of crap – acknowledge it and change. Once you break out of your old thinking you'll be amazed at how you can turn things around.
www.manvfat.com/members/admin

RECIPES

The recipes given in this section are to give a more detailed indication of what you might eat each day on any given diet. You should consider that these recipes are largely to give you a general idea of the types of foods that fit with different diets. If you are looking to research more varied diets then take a look at www.manvfat.com/diets

All recipes serve one unless otherwise stated. All calorie values are approximate.

MY OWN RULES

BREAKFAST HOMEMADE MUESLI
(Makes 13 servings)

Ingredients
225g (8oz) oats
100g (3½oz) mixed nuts (such as almonds, macadamias or walnuts)
20g (¾oz) dried goji berries
120g (4oz) mixed seeds (such as linseeds, sunflower, chai seeds or sesame seeds)
160g (5¾oz) mixed dried fruit (such as raisins, apricots or cranberries)
a handful of coconut chips (optional)

Method
1. Mix all of the ingredients together and put in an airtight container.
2. Feel smug that you've just sorted out breakfast for the next 13 days.
3. For one serving, weigh out 50g (2oz) of muesli and add 100ml (3½fl oz) full-fat milk and a handful of fresh berries.

LUNCH HAM AND EGG SALAD

Salads are actually considerably more exciting than they sound, provided you experiment with combinations. You need to learn how to build a salad – it's an art, so get creative and enjoy it.

There are a five stages to making a great salad:

1. Choose a leafy base (lettuce, spinach, etc).
2. Add some brightly coloured salad items (e.g. tomatoes, cucumber, peppers, beetroot).
3. Add protein (chicken, ham, boiled egg, tuna, grilled tofu, cheese, avocado).
4. Choose a dressing.
5. Add a handful of nuts/ seeds.

The combinations are endless but this one should get you started.

Method
1. Prepare your leafy base – a mixture of watercress and rocket leaves works well for this particular one.
2. Chop up your brightly coloured salad items – 1 stick of celery, half a red pepper, a couple of tomatoes, a few slices of cucumber and half a red onion.
3. Add your protein – 80g (3oz) of sliced ham and a peeled boiled egg, cut in half.
4. Make up your dressing – mix together 1 tablespoon of balsamic vinegar with 3 tablespoons of olive oil, a teaspoon of Dijon mustard and half a crushed garlic clove. Drizzle over your salad.
5. Add nuts/seeds – in this case, scatter over a handful of pumpkin seeds.

DINNER THAI GREEN CURRY WITH CHICKEN
(Serves 4)

Ingredients
1 tablespoon coconut oil
2 garlic cloves, crushed
1 thumbsize piece of fresh ginger, peeled and finely chopped
1 tablespoon Thai green curry paste
   (or red, depending on how spicy you like your curry)
1 x 400ml (14fl oz) tin light coconut milk
400g (14oz) chicken breasts, cut into bite-sized chunks
1 aubergine, sliced
1 teaspoon fish sauce
300g (10½oz) brown rice
handful of coriander leaves, to serve
juice of ½ lime, to serve

Method
1. Heat the coconut oil in a pan over a medium heat, add the garlic and ginger and fry for 1–2 minutes.
2. Add the curry paste and give everything a quick stir, then pour in the coconut milk and bring to a simmer.
3. Add the chicken breast chunks, aubergine slices and fish sauce and leave to simmer for about 15 minutes, stirring occasionally, until the chicken is cooked.
4. While the curry is simmering, cook the rice according to the packet instructions.
5. Divide the rice between bowls, spoon over the curry and top with the coriander leaves and lime juice.

 The chicken can be substituted with 400g (14oz) beef or prawns, or 300g (10½oz) tofu.

CALORIE COUNTING FOR A DAY OF 1200 CALORIES

BREAKFAST PORRIDGE
(350 calories)

This is a good simple porridge recipe that can be tweaked depending on your diet – to increase the calorie count add a handful of seeds before serving (chai seeds are packed with nutrients and will keep you fuller for longer), while to reduce the calories use more water and less milk.

Ingredients
50g (2oz) porridge oats
150ml (¼ pint) skimmed milk
150ml (¼ pint) water
handful of berries (blueberries, strawberries or raspberries)
1 teaspoon honey

Method
1. Mix the oats, milk and water together in a pan, bring to a simmer and cook for around 5 minutes, stirring until thick and creamy.
2. Spoon into a bowl, top with berries and drizzle over the honey to finish.

To power up this porridge, use jumbo organic oats if possible, and soak them (this will allow them to be more easily digested) the night before in water along with a handful of goji berries (¼ cup = 90 calories). If you can, try to get hold of local raw honey – as well as tasting better than the regular shop-bought stuff it has been suggested that it combats hayfever and seasonal allergies.

LUNCH MACKEREL AND RICE
(356 calories)

Ingredients
75g (2½oz) brown rice
1 x 140g (4½oz) fillet of ready-to-eat
   smoked mackerel, shredded
100g (3½oz) cooked beetroot, cubed

Method
1. Cook the rice according to packet instructions.
2. When the rice is cooked and has been drained, add the mackerel and beetroot and mix.

For an even speedier version of this recipe you can use the one minute microwave rice and stock up on tinned mackerel, which lasts for ages so is a good store-cupboard ingredient. Try the tinned mackerel in tomato sauce to vary the recipe (it'll only be an extra 40 calories).

DINNER CHILLI CON CARNE
(Serves 3 – 490 calories per portion)

Ingredients

1 tablespoon olive oil
1 onion, chopped
500g (1lb) lean minced beef
1 beef stock cube
1 teaspoon chilli powder
1 teaspoon ground cumin
2 x 400g (14oz) tins chopped tomatoes
1 x 400g (14oz) tin kidney beans, drained
1 x 400g (14oz) tin black-eyed beans, drained

Method

1. Heat the oil in a pan over a medium heat, add the onion and minced beef and cook, stirring regularly, until browned.
2. Add the stock cube, chilli powder and cumin, along with the chopped tomatoes.
3. Stir in the kidney and black-eyed beans, bring to a simmer and leave to cook, stirring occasionally, for at least an hour, until the sauce has thickened and the flavours have combined.

TIP *This chilli is great cooked in the slow cooker – as well as tasting so much better it breaks the food down more, making it much easier to digest. Pop it on before you go out in the morning and it will be ready when you get home.*

5:2 FASTING DAY

BREAKFAST BOILED EGGS AND ASPARAGUS
(182 calories)

Ingredients

2 eggs
100g (3½oz) asparagus tips
salt

Method

1. Carefully add your eggs to a pan of boiling water and cook to your liking (like tea, this is a very individual taste, and you need to experiment to work out your egg sweet spot –

between 3 minutes for soft-boiled to 7 minutes for hard-boiled).

2. Before the eggs have finished cooking, add the asparagus tips to the pan and cook for 3–5 minutes until soft but not limp. Drain.

3. Season the eggs with a little salt and enjoy by dipping them with the asparagus.

LUNCH MISO SOUP

(Serves 3 – 175 calories per serving)

Ingredients
low-calorie cooking spray
2 spring onions, sliced
1 tablespoon miso paste
420ml (15fl oz) boiling water
1 vegetable or fish stock cube
300g (10½oz) tofu, cut into cubes
pinch of dried seaweed

Method
1. Spray the bottom of a pan with cooking spray, add the spring onions and fry for 2–3 minutes until softened. Stir in the miso paste and cook, stirring for 1 minute.

2. Pour over the water, add the stock cube and stir together well to dissolve.

3. Add the tofu and seaweed, bring to a simmer and cook for around 5 minutes. Serve.

DINNER COD FILLET AND CAULIFLOWER

(295 calories)

Ingredients
4 cauliflower florets
1 small potato, peeled
1 x 140g (5oz) cod fillet
salt and pepper
pinch of chilli flakes (optional)
low-calorie cooking spray

Method
1. Chop the cauliflower and potato into even bite-size pieces. Boil the potato for 15–20 minutes until soft and either boil or steam the cauliflower for 5–10 minutes until tender.

2. Season the cod with salt and pepper and sprinkle with chilli flakes if you like a bit of spice. Spray the bottom of a griddle pan with low-calorie cooking spray and set over a high heat. Add the cod and fry for around 3 minutes on each side until cooked.

LOW-CARB, HIGH-FAT

BREAKFAST HEALTHY FRY-UP

Ingredients
1 tablespoon butter
1 sausage
2 bacon rashers
1 egg
a handful of
mushrooms, sliced
2 large tomatoes,
halved

Method
1. Melt the butter in a large frying pan over a medium heat, add the sausage and cook, turning occasionally, for 10–12 minutes until browned on all sides.
2. Add the bacon to the pan and fry for a couple of minutes longer.
3. Crack the egg into the pan, add the mushrooms and tomatoes, and cook for a further 3–4 minutes until the egg is cooked to your liking and the mushrooms and tomatoes are soft. Serve.

LUNCH GREEK SALAD
(Serves 3)

It's good to have leftovers of this salad as it goes really well with lots of other dishes. If you're using a fresh lemon for the juice, chuck a few of the leftover wedges into a large jug of cold filtered water to make a refreshing drink.

Ingredients
1 iceburg lettuce, washed and sliced
1 cucumber, sliced
1 red onion, sliced
4 large vine tomatoes, cut into quarters
100g (3½oz) black olives
200g (7oz) feta cheese, cubed
1 tablespoon lemon juice
3 tablespoons olive oil

Method
1. Mix together the lettuce, cucumber, onion and tomatoes in a bowl.
2. Top with the olives and feta cheese.
3. Make the dressing by mixing together the lemon juice and olive oil. Drizzle over the salad to finish.

DINNER LAMB STEAK WITH YOGURT AND HARISSA

These steaks are great served with the leftover salad from lunch.

Ingredients
1 tablespoon olive oil
1 garlic clove, peeled
  and crushed
1 x 80g (3oz) lamb steak
5g (¼oz) pine nuts
3 tablespoons
  full-fat yogurt
1 tablespoon
  harissa paste

Method
1. Heat the oil in a griddle pan over a medium heat, add the garlic and fry for 1–2 minutes until lightly browned.
2. Add the lamb steak and fry until cooked to your liking (around 5–6 minutes on each side for medium). Remove from the pan and set aside to rest.
3. Add the pine nuts to the pan and toast for a couple of minutes until lightly golden.
4. Mix the yogurt together with the harissa and serve with the lamb steak, scattering over the pine nuts to finish.

PALEO

BREAKFAST EGGS AND SPINACH

Ingredients
2 eggs
salt and pepper
120g (4oz) spinach
  leaves, washed
  and dried
1 tablespoon coconut oil

Method
1. Crack the eggs into a mixing bowl, season with salt and pepper and whisk together well.
2. Add the spinach and mix together again.
3. Heat the coconut oil in a non-stick frying pan over a medium heat. Add the egg and spinach mixture and stir occasionally to scramble (which means mixing every ten seconds or so until the eggs are set but a bit soft in places). Serve.

 TIP *You can add some bacon or other meat/fish to this if you want a bigger breakfast.*

LUNCH BAKED SWEET POTATO WITH BACON AND MUSHROOMS

Ingredients

1 large sweet potato
2 tablespoons olive oil
pinch of salt
2 bacon rashers
a handful of mushrooms
2 teaspoons coconut oil

Method

1. Wash the sweet potato and prick all over with a fork. Leave to dry and then rub with 1 tablespoon of olive oil and a pinch of salt.

2. Place in a cold oven and switch on to 170°C/335°F/ Gas 3½. Bake for 1½ hours, until the baked potato is soft when pricked with a fork.

3. 10 minutes before serving, heat the remaining olive oil in a pan, add the bacon and mushrooms and fry until golden and cooked.

4. Split the baked potato in half and spoon over the coconut oil. Serve with the bacon and mushrooms.

DINNER ROAST CHICKEN WITH ROAST VEGETABLES
(Serves 4)

Ingredients

2 onions
1 lemon
1 x 2kg (4lb)
   chicken
2 garlic cloves
1 tablespoon
   olive oil
½ x Roast
   Vegetables
   (see page 231),
   to serve

Method

1. Preheat the oven to 190°C/375°F/Gas 5.

2. Cut the onions in half and lay on a roasting tray.

3. Cut the lemon into wedges and stuff into the chicken.

4. Crush the garlic cloves and rub over the chicken along with the olive oil.

5. Put the chicken on top of the onions and roast for 1 hour and 45 minutes, increasing the heat to 220°C/425°F/Gas 7 for the last 15 minutes for a crispy skin. Baste (coat the chicken with its juices) a couple of times during roasting. You can tell when the chicken is cooked by piercing the part between the leg and the body; the juices should run clear. Allow the chicken to rest for 30 minutes before serving.

6. Serve with roast vegetables or steamed broccoli and peas.

WEIGHT WATCHERS

These are examples of what you would eat on a normal Weight Watchers day, but you should check quantities with your own Weight Watchers allowances and plan.

BREAKFAST BEANS ON TOAST

Ingredients
200g (7oz) baked beans
2 slices wholemeal bread
1 tablespoon low-fat
   spread

Method
1. Heat the baked beans in a small pan until warm.
2. Toast your bread, spread with low-fat spread and top with the baked beans.
3. Tuck in.

LUNCH HALLOUMI AND SPINACH WITH BEETROOT

As vegetables are free on the Weight Watchers plan feel free to increase the amount of spinach and beetroot in this recipe.

Ingredients
1 teaspoon olive oil
75g (2½oz) halloumi
   cheese, sliced
100g (3½oz) spinach leaves
50g (2oz) cooked beetroot,
   cut into slices

Method
1. Heat the olive oil in griddle or frying pan over a medium heat, add the halloumi cheese and cook for 2 minutes.
2. Add the spinach and fry for a further few minutes until the cheese has a golden look to it and the spinach is cooked.
3. Serve with the cooked beetroot.

DINNER HOMEMADE FISH AND CHIPS

Ingredients

2 potatoes
1 tablespoon olive oil
salt
1 x 140g (4½oz) salmon fillet
1 garlic clove, crushed
2 lemon slices
broccoli, cut into florets, to serve

Method

1. Heat the oven to 200°C/400°F/Gas 6.

2. Make the chips first – simply scrub and clean the potatoes (or peel), and slice into even chip-sized pieces. Put them in boiling water for 2–3 minutes, drain and place on a baking tray. Drizzle with half the olive oil, sprinkle with salt and cook in the oven for about 45 minutes or until golden.

3. While the chips are cooking, place the salmon on a large piece of tin foil, drizzle with the remaining olive oil and top with the crushed garlic and lemon slices. Wrap up into a parcel and bake in the oven for 15–20 minutes until cooked.

4. Serve with as much steamed broccoli as you like.

 TIP *You can use sweet potatoes or other root veg (e.g. beetroot, carrots) instead of potatoes to make the chips.*

SLIMMING WORLD

These are examples of what you would eat on a normal Slimming World day, but you should check quantities with your own Slimming World allowances and plan.

BREAKFAST TAKE-AWAY YOGURT AND GRANOLA BREAKFAST

Ingredients

150g (5oz) fat-free Greek yogurt
35g (1oz) oats
50g (2oz) berries (such as raspberries, strawberries or blueberries)

Method

1. Pop the yogurt into a jam jar or Tupperware bowl.

2. Top with the oats and berries, seal and take with you to enjoy later.

 TIP *Try and get hold of live yogurt to boost your good bacteria (see page 141 for information on probiotics).*

LUNCH COUSCOUS SALAD WITH ROASTED VEGETABLES
(Serves 2 with leftover vegetables)

Ingredients

150g (5oz) couscous
juice of 1 lemon
salt and pepper

Roasted Vegetables

6 tomatoes
1 red pepper
1 yellow pepper
1 red onion
1 aubergine
low-calorie cooking spray
2 garlic cloves, crushed

Method

1. Preheat the oven to 200°C/400°F/Gas 6.

2. For the roasted vegetables, chop all the veg into even bite-sized pieces and spread them out over a large baking tray. Spray with a little of the cooking spray and spoon over the garlic.

3. Roast in the oven for around 30 minutes, until the vegetables are lightly golden and cooked through.

4. Meanwhile, prepare the couscous. Put it in a bowl, squeeze over the lemon juice and season with salt and pepper. Pour over 175ml (6fl oz) boiling water, cover the bowl with clingfilm and leave for 5 minutes, stirring occasionally, until the grains are soft and the water has been absorbed.

5. Spoon half the vegetables into the couscous, mix together and serve.

DINNER CHICKEN AND PESTO PASTA

This recipe makes more pesto than you need for the pasta, so you could increase the pasta and chicken portions and make enough for lunch the next day. It's also very good served with the leftover roast vegetables from lunch.

Ingredients

100g (3oz) skinless chicken
   breast, cut into strips
low-calorie cooking spray
1 bunch of fresh basil leaves
50g (2oz) Parmesan, grated
2 garlic cloves
100g (3½oz) fat-free
   fromage frais
100ml (3½fl oz) vegetable
   stock
a handful of fresh parsley
100g (3½oz) wholemeal
   pasta

Method

1. Gently fry the chicken strips in a little of the low-calorie spray oil for 8–12 minutes until cooked through.
2. To make the pesto, add the basil leaves, Parmesan, garlic cloves, fromage frais, vegetable stock and parsley to a blender and blitz. Set aside.
3. Meanwhile, cook the pasta in a pan of boiling water according to the packet instructions. Drain.
4. Stir the chicken strips and 1–2 tablespoons of pesto through the pasta and serve.

JUICE DETOX

BREAKFAST THE ORANGE ONE

Ingredients
2 apples
4 carrots
1 thumbsize piece of
    ginger (optional)

Method
1. Wash your apples and carrots and peel your ginger, if using. Add the ingredients to the juicer, remembering to put the ginger in the middle of the apples and carrots so it gets pushed through properly.

LUNCH THE GREEN ONE

Ingredients
1 lemon or lime,
    unwaxed if possible
2 apples
1 cucumber
a handful of spinach leaves
a handful of kale leaves
2 sticks celery
4 broccoli florets

Method
1. If you are able to get hold of an unwaxed lemon or lime you can use it whole, otherwise peel it.
2. Wash all the ingredients, chopping them where necessary so they fit into the juicer.
3. Juice and enjoy.

DINNER THE RED ONE

Ingredients
1 thumbsize piece of ginger
1 lemon or lime,
    unwaxed if possible
2 raw beetroots
1 cucumber
2 apples
a handful of kale or
    spinach leaves

Method
1. Peel the ginger. If you are able to get hold of an unwaxed lemon or lime you can use it whole, otherwise peel it.
2. Wash all the ingredients, chopping them where necessary so they fit into the juicer.
3. Juice and enjoy.

SLOW CARB DIET

BREAKFAST OMELETTE

Ingredients
1 tablespoon olive oil
1–2 bacon rashers
2 eggs
salt and pepper
70g (3oz) mushrooms,
  thinly sliced

Method
1. Heat the oil over a medium heat, add the bacon and fry until cooked. Remove from the pan and set aside.
2. Whisk the eggs together in a bowl and season with salt and pepper. Add the mushroom slices and mix well.
3. Add the egg and mushroom mix to the pan and cook until the eggs are setting but still slightly runny, around 1–2 minutes.
4. Add the bacon slices and cook for a further 1–2 minutes until the omelette is set firm.

LUNCH BEEF STEW
(Serves 4)

Ingredients
1 turnip or swede
2 carrots
1 onion
2 sticks celery
450g (14½oz) braising
  steak, cubed
1 tablespoon coconut oil
1 beef stock cube
2 large tomatoes,
  skinned
80g (3oz) red lentils

Method
1. Peel and chop the turnip, carrots, onion and celery into bite-sized pieces.
2. Throw the steak and the vegetables into a pan with the coconut oil and fry for a few minutes, stirring regularly, until the beef is browned on all sides.
3. Make up the beef stock by mixing the stock cube with 500ml (17fl oz) boiling water.
4. Add the tomatoes and lentils to the pan, pour over the stock and bring to a simmer. Cook over a gentle heat, uncovered, for at least an hour, until the stew has thickened and the beef, lentils and vegetables are soft.

This is a great one to do in a big batch and freeze in individual portions. It cooks well in a slow cooker.

DINNER PRAWN STIR-FRY
(Serves 4)

Ingredients
1 tablespoon sesame oil
2 garlic cloves, crushed
1 thumbsize piece of ginger, peeled and finely sliced
1 fresh chilli, finely chopped
400g (14oz) cooked king prawns
1 bunch of spring onions, chopped
100g (3½oz) beansprouts
1 red pepper, sliced
100g (3½oz) green beans, chopped
2 tablespoons soy sauce

Method
1. Heat the sesame oil in a frying pan or wok, add the garlic, ginger and chilli and stir-fry for 1–2 minutes.
2. Add the prawns and stir-fry for a further 1–2 minutes, then add the spring onions, beansprouts, pepper and green beans and soy sauce and stir-fry for 2–3 minutes until the ingredients are cooked.

The prawns can be replaced with chicken or beef. If you would like a spicier version you can add a teaspoon of dried chilli flakes as well.

DRINKS

WATER

Yes, health professionals do harp on about this but it's so good for you! Interestingly, the weight-loss benefits of water are under scrutiny, but the litmus test with the eight glasses per day rule is to try it yourself and see if you feel healthier. If you can drink it with a wedge of lemon or lime it makes it a bit more interesting and adds a healthy angle – citric acid in lemon and lime is immune boosting and anti-bacterial. Read more about the benefits of filtering your water and consider purchasing a water filter.

COCONUT WATER

Great for hydration, this is an isotonic drink (so it has a similar level of salt and sugar as in the human body) that has no sugar but tastes sweet and is very refreshing, especially when chilled.

HERBAL TEA

Herbal teas are a healthy alternative to caffeinated hot drinks, and a great way to get a gentle burst of nourishing herbs into your system. There are so many flavours on the market that it's worth trying a few to find some that you like.

KOMBUCHA

Kombucha is a fermented probiotic tea drink with a taste that takes a while to get used to. It's a mixture of sugar, tea, bacteria and yeast, and is rich in antioxidants and vitamins. It also contains organic acids and is a probiotic, so helps to maintain a strong digestive system.

MILK

A great source of calcium which helps regulate muscle contractions including heartbeat. An adult needs 700mg of calcium per day and a 250ml glass of 1% fat milk gives you 300mg. If you are interested in unpasteurised food take a look at the options locally for raw milk, at www.realmilk.com.

KEFIR

Kefir grains are a combination of bacteria and yeasts and to make the drink the grains are placed in milk and left to ferment. It is packed with probiotics and is fantastic for your digestive system and, consequently, your immune system. You can buy a starter pack to make your own kefir or buy it ready-made. It tastes like slightly fizzy yogurt, which isn't exactly appealing (certainly at first), so drink it chilled, add cinnamon or honey to it or, better yet, add it to a smoothie.

INDEX

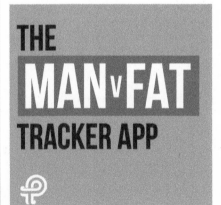